CONTENTS

THE COMPLETE GUIDE TO
PERSONAL TRAINING

Morc Coulson

B L O O M S B U R Y
LONDON • NEW DELHI • NEW YORK • SYDNEY

Note

Whilst every effort has been made to ensure that the content of this book is as technically accurate and as sound as possible, neither the author nor the publishers can accept responsibility for any injury or loss sustained as a result of the use of this material.

Published by Bloomsbury Publishing Plc
50 Bedford Square
London WC1B 3DP
www.bloomsbury.com

First edition 2013

Copyright © 2013 Morc Coulson

ISBN (print): 978 1 4081 8723 4
ISBN (Epub): 978 1 4081 9630 4
ISBN (Epdf): 978 1 4081 9631 1

SkillsActive is proud to endorse *The Complete Guide to Personal Training*. This book, through its offering of expert advice and guidance, supports our mission to get 'More People. Better Skilled. Better Qualified'.

SkillsActive is the Sector Skills Council for Active Leisure, Learning and Well-being and works to increase the demand, quality and availability of skills provision across the UK.

SkillsActive's nationwide body of staff are experts in their field. They provide employers, training providers, policy makers and key organisations with information and advice on skills development and training for the sector.

By reading this book, REPs registered Fitness Professional will achieve 3 CPD points. Find out more at www.skillsactive.com

A CIP catalogue record for this book is available from the British Library.

Acknowledgements
Cover photograph © Shutterstock
Inside photographs © Chris Heron with the exception of the following; pp. 21, 65 and 155 (bottom) © Shutterstock
Illustrations by David Gardner
Designed by James Watson
Commissioned by Charlotte Croft
Edited by Sarah Cole

This book is produced using paper that is made from wood grown in managed, sustainable forests. It is natural, renewable and recyclable. The logging and manufacturing processes conform to the environmental regulations of the country of origin.

Typeset in 10.75pt on 14pt Adobe Caslon by seagulls.net

Printed and bound in China by C&C Offset Printing Co. Ltd

10 9 8 7 6 5 4 3

ABOUT THIS BOOK

PART ONE
THE FOUNDATIONS OF PERSONAL TRAINING

This section outlines the structure of the health and fitness industry and discusses the role of the instructor in relation to codes of conduct and client care. This section also investigates the role of reflective practice to identify strengths and weaknesses in order to put in place appropriate strategies for continuing professional development.

PART TWO
PLAN EXERCISE PROGRAMMES

This section looks at the ways in which instructors gather their clients' information during the screening process and how to analyse them, using behavioural, physiological and psychological parameters. This section also discusses how to design exercise programmes for healthy adults of all ages (this may include young people in the 14–16 age range, provided they are part of a larger adult group) using the information collected.

PART THREE
DELIVER EXERCISE PROGRAMMES

This section is related to the skills that personal trainers require to teach exercise programmes to healthy adults of all ages (this may include young people in the 14–16 age range, provided they are part of a larger adult group) using appropriate teaching and motivational styles. This section also covers giving appropriate client feedback using a variety of communication methods in order to improve client understanding of all aspects of the exercise programme.

PART FOUR
MANAGING EXERCISE PROGRAMMES

This section is related to the skills that personal trainers require to manage, review and adapt exercise programmes for apparently healthy adults of all ages (this may include young people in the 14–16 age range, provided they are part of a larger adult group) using effective communication and feedback methods. This section also discusses various training methods and provides a range of useful exercise techniques appropriate for personal training.

PART FIVE
SPECIAL POPULATIONS AND EXERCISE

This section outlines the life-cycle of the musculoskeletal system (including bone) and its implications for working with special populations including 14–16 year old young people, disabled people, older people (50+) and ante- and postnatal women. This section also deals with the contraindications and key safety guidelines when delivering exercise programmes to special populations.

PART SIX
NUTRITION, EXERCISE AND WEIGHT MANAGEMENT

This section explores how nutrition can affect a person's general health as well as physical performance. It also explores links between diet and physical activity and their combined role in optimum health and wellbeing. This section also discusses nutrition and its relationship to physical activity and exercise so that the personal trainer can provide safe and appropriate nutritional advice to clients taking into account national guidelines on nutrition. Finally, this section highlights the professional role boundaries when applying the principles of nutrition in the context of safe professional practice.

PART SEVEN
HEALTH AND SAFETY IN PRACTICE

This section explores regulations and statutory frameworks relating to the health and safety of customers, colleagues and trainers. This section also covers the identification of hazards, assessing and controlling risks as they occur and dealing with incidents and emergencies. Finally, this section also has an important element on safeguarding children and other vulnerable people.

PART EIGHT
SALES AND MARKETING IN PRACTICE

This section deals with how to identify potential clients using market research techniques and how to advertise your services. Selling is an integral part of the marketing process, and this is also dealt with in this section. Finally, this section deals with financial management systems relevant to the self-employed or employed personal trainer.

INTRODUCTION

Human beings have evolved over millions of years into hunter-gatherers, and genetically we have changed only a fraction since then. Essentially, our bodies are adapted to a hunter-gatherer existence which back then required high levels of energy for activities such as building shelters and fires, gathering food and water, tracking and hunting. In current times, however, activity levels are much different as people spend much of their lives using labour-saving devices, and many jobs involve sitting down at a computer all day. This leads to sedentary behaviour, which combined with poor nutritional habits is leading to an ever-increasing obese population. Many people these days don't know how to exercise properly – which can lead to injury – or they need help to keep motivated and this is where the personal trainer can help.

Let's first distinguish between sedentary and inactive behaviour. Inactive can be used to describe those individuals who do not meet the physical activity guidelines for moderate and vigorous physical activity but they might not be classed as sedentary. On the other hand, an adult or child who is physically active can still be considered sedentary if they spend a large amount of time doing any of the following behaviours:

- sitting while at work or school
- watching television
- using a computer or playing video games – this excludes 'active' gaming such as Wii or X-box Kinect which requires whole-body movement.
- reading
- sitting while socialising with friends or family
- sitting in a car or other form of motorised transport – for a young child, this could include being carried in a car seat or pushed in a buggy.

It can be seen that according to the Sedentary Behaviour Research Network (2012) this is a group of behaviours that occur while sitting or lying down and that require very low energy

Table 0.1	Health risks associated with sedentary behaviour in adults and children
Adults (health risks)	**Children (health risks)**
<ul><li>type 2 diabetes</li><li>cardiovascular disease</li><li>metabolic syndrome</li><li>death from all causes</li><li>emerging evidence for depression</li><li>possible risk of certain cancers</li></ul>	<ul><li>lower levels of aerobic fitness</li><li>risk of cardiovascular disease</li><li>overweight/obesity – but as with adults the evidence is weak as calorie intake often contributes</li><li>emerging link to mental health</li><li>developing sedentary habits into adulthood</li></ul>

expenditure. There is concern that sedentary behaviour is leading to an increase in health complications. For example, according to the British Heart Foundation (2012), research shows that sedentary behaviour is associated with increased health risks for both adults and children as shown in table 0.1

Although the link between sedentary behaviour and health risks have been acknowledged for some time, the levels of sedentary behaviour in adults and children have been increasing steadily over the years. There are many possible reasons for this, however, the general public's lack of information, or not understanding exactly what is meant by sedentary behaviour, could well be an important factor. For this reason, the trainer should identify education as a main priority when working with clients with a view to fostering lifestyle changes that will hopefully result in an increase in public awareness. In terms of levels and types of sedentary behaviour in the UK, the Health Survey for England (2009) report provides information across a range of age groups as can be seen in figures 0.1 to 0.6.

SEDENTARY BEHAVIOUR OF CHILDREN IN ENGLAND

The report includes information relating to the sedentary behaviour of children in England. It shows that as children grow older they generally spend more time being sedentary. The report states that 4–7 year olds spend 6–7 hours per day being sedentary whereas 12–15 year olds spend 8–9 hours per day being sedentary. When sedentary behaviour was analysed further it showed that 41% of boys and 13% of girls reported more than two hours of computer console use per day. It was also reported that children (aged 2 to 15) in England watch more TV on weekend days than weekdays as shown in figure 0.1.

SEDENTARY BEHAVIOUR OF CHILDREN IN WALES

The Health Survey report also provides information relating to the sedentary behaviour of children in Wales. Figure 0.2 outlines the main findings relating to screen viewing for ages 12 to 16 which are as follows:

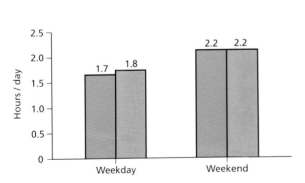

Figure 0.1 TV viewing in English children aged 2–15 years (blue: boys, red: girls)

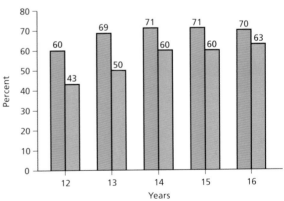

Figure 0.2 Proportion of Welsh children exceeding 2 hours per day screen viewing (blue: TV, red: computer)

- 60% of 12 year olds reported ≥ 2 hours of TV viewing and 43% reported ≥ 2 hours of computer usage.
- TV use peaked between 14 and 15 year olds with 71% ≥ 2 hours of use whereas computer use peaked with 16 years old at 63%.

The report also shows that on average for children aged 11–16 years old:

- 67% of girls and 70% of boys reported > 2 hours TV viewing on a weekday.
- 61% of girls and 51% of boys reported > 2 computer usage on a weekday.

SEDENTARY BEHAVIOUR OF CHILDREN IN NORTHERN IRELAND

According to the report it can be seen from the information in figure 0.3 that the largest proportion of young people in Northern Ireland, aged 11–16 years, reported using the TV or computer/console games up to 10 hours per week with a considerable proportion for more than 10 hours

per week. Only 4% of children reported watching no TV.

SEDENTARY BEHAVIOUR OF CHILDREN IN SCOTLAND

The Health Survey reported the following information relating to the sedentary behaviour of children in Scotland (see figure 0.4):

- 30% of children approximately four years old exceeded two hours of TV viewing per day.
- By age 11, 62% of boys and 57% of girls exceed two hours of TV viewing (weekday).
- By age 15, 69% of boys and 68% of girls exceed two hours of TV viewing (weekday).
- 53% of boys and 29% of girls aged 11 years reported more than two hours of computer game play alone (weekdays). At age 15 years, it increased to 64% in boys but decreased to 26% in girls.

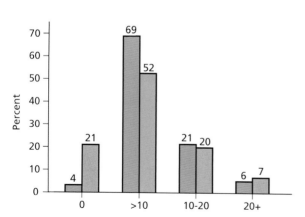

Figure 0.3 Hours of use per week in young children in Northern Ireland (blue: TV, red: computer)

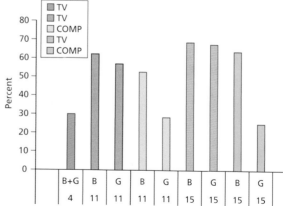

Figure 0.4 Proportion of Scottish children exceeding 2 hours per day screen viewing

SEDENTARY BEHAVIOUR OF ADULTS IN ENGLAND

It can be seen from figure 0.5 that information from the Health Survey relating to the sedentary behaviour of adults in England is as follows:

- Between the ages of 16–64, sedentary time remains relatively stable with both men and women averaging about 9.5 hours of sedentary time.
- Between the ages of 65–74, sedentary time for both men and women increased to 10 hours per day or more.
- By age 75+ years, individuals were sedentary for 11 hours per day.

SEDENTARY BEHAVIOUR OF ADULTS IN SCOTLAND

It can be seen from figure 0.6 that information on the sedentary behaviour of adults in Scotland in relation to TV and other screen viewing is as follows:

- Overall, the largest proportion of adults (34%) spent > 4 hours a day on screen activities.

- 21% of adults spent 3-4 hours per day on screen based activities.
- 28% of adults spent 2–3 hours per day on screen based activities.
- Only 17% of adults spent less than 2 hours per day on screen based activities.

The report also stated that on average men spend 3.6 hours and women spend 3.2 hours on TV viewing and other screen based activities per day.

The information from the Health Survey for England report highlights the increasing problem of sedentary behaviour in the UK, especially in view of the overwhelming evidence to show that regular physical activity can help to reduce the incidence of many chronic conditions that are caused by sedentary behaviour by up to 50%. For example, the physiological and psychological benefits of a physically active lifestyle are well documented in public health guidelines such as those published by the Department of Health (2011). It should be mentioned, however, that some individuals might meet recommended daily levels of physical activity but might also incorporate prolonged bouts of

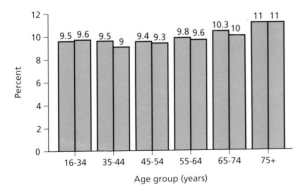

Figure 0.5 Total sedentary time in English adults (blue: men, red: women)

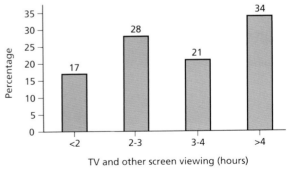

Figure 0.6 Daily TV and other screen viewing in Scottish adults

sedentary behaviour into their daily lifestyles. For this reason one of the main roles of the personal trainer (from here on referred to as the trainer or PT) is to help facilitate individuals to make the transition to a healthier and more active *lifestyle* rather than just focus on specific individual exercise sessions.

PERSONAL TRAINER VALUES

Advertising, magazines, newspapers, films and TV constantly bombard us with powerful images of the 'ideal body', which is often linked with success and wealth. As trainers we should know that only a very small percentage of the population are genetically disposed to look like that. It is the role of the health and fitness industry to educate people to value all kinds of body types, so that people can have a healthy body while not trying to conform to an impossible ideal. The health and fitness industry, and those people working in it, first need to ensure that trainers are seen as the professionals they are. Too often PTs are perceived by the public as doing little other than count backwards from 10 reps, a kind of supercharged training buddy. However, most PTs dedicate much time and effort to their profession and continuing development and as such should be acknowledged and rewarded accordingly. The main purpose of this book is twofold: firstly, to provide a comprehensive text for potential personal trainers which covers all of the relevant criteria of the National Occupational Standards. Secondly, it is to enthuse qualified PTs to further develop and maintain the professionalism of the industry by using the tools in this book. Whether qualified or not, the 5 Es, which is reflected throughout the entire content of this book, is a set of values that all trainers should aspire to:

- Empathise: this is a crucial quality for trainers. By empathising with clients, the chances of a successful relationship with them are greatly increased.
- Encourage: trainers should always encourage clients to adopt healthy lifestyles and not just focus on the time spent with them.
- Evaluate: constantly evaluate and re-evaluate lifestyle programmes as circumstances often change.
- Empower: trying to empower clients to take responsibility for their own lifestyle is one of the main aims of the trainer, which is evident in the Code of Conduct.
- Evolve: regularly reflect on yourself as a personal trainer in terms of your own self-development and the development of your business product.

PART ONE
THE FOUNDATIONS OF PERSONAL TRAINING

PROFESSIONAL PRACTICE

1

THE NATIONAL OCCUPATIONAL STANDARDS (NOS) LEVEL 3 PERSONAL TRAINER CRITERIA COVERED IN THIS CHAPTER ARE:

- The values or codes of practice relevant to the work you are carrying out and their importance
- The role of the fitness professional in the industry and the structure of the industry
- The importance of reflection and continuing professional development in helping to develop client fitness and motivation
- Industry organisations and their relevance to the fitness professional
- Appropriate registration systems and continuing professional development requirements
- Employment opportunities in different sectors of the industry
- The difference between advising on exercise participation and lifestyle physical activity
- How to present a positive image of yourself and your organisation
- Why the relationship based on trust and openness between the instructor and client is important
- The type of instructor/client relationship which will assist client progress and adherence to physical activity
- The types of personal qualities that instructors need to develop in order to help and support clients
- Why your clients need to understand your role and responsibilities and the roles and responsibilities of other professionals
- The extent/ limitations of your own role and responsibility when working with clients
- What is meant by a 'professional relationship' between instructor and client
- What is meant by 'valuing diversity' in a practical context when working with clients
- The types of prejudice and discrimination that individual clients might experience and how to overcome these
- What is meant by 'confidentiality' and why it is important when working with clients, other staff and professionals
- The types of information that may be covered by confidentiality agreements
- How to maintain confidentiality

- How to manage conflict and disagreements with colleagues
- Procedures to follow in the event of client complaints
- How to establish rapport with your clients and the communication skills you need

THE INDUSTRY

The health and fitness sector is made up of both private (commercial) and public providers (such as local authority leisure centres) and has grown substantially over the years to a club membership of almost 5 million (mainly in the private sector). This figure can be misleading, however, as there are many public-sector participants but on a pay-as-you-go basis. A number of leading chains have developed with less and less 'stand alone' clubs across the sector. There appears to have been a shift in focus over the years from physical fitness to health and wellbeing. This shift was emphasised in 2007 when Nuffield (a health care company in the UK) took over Cannons Health and Fitness Clubs. It is also emphasised by the additional services offered by clubs including physiotherapy, massage, relaxation, clinics and homeopathy, etc.

However, despite the high club membership across the public and private sectors, it is becoming increasingly more difficult to gain employment in the health and fitness industry (referred to from now on as just 'the industry'), especially for those individuals who do not possess appropriate qualifications. In order to aid individuals in this process and help make the industry more professional, organisations such as the Fitness Industry Association (FIA) and SkillsActive have taken a lead role. The FIA was founded in 1991 to drive up participation and address concerns in the industry relating to safety and unfair codes of conduct. The FIA now works closely with government to help

deliver its public health targets and represent the interests of health and fitness organisations across the United Kingdom. FIA members include operators from the public and private sector, service/product suppliers to the industry, training providers, independent professionals and affiliated bodies. SkillsActive is licensed by government as the Sector Skills Council for Active Leisure and Wellbeing. Charged by employers, SkillsActive leads the skills and productivity drive across the sport and recreation, health and fitness, outdoors, playwork, and caravan industries – known as the active leisure and learning sector. SkillsActive works with health and fitness professionals across the United Kingdom to ensure the workforce is appropriately skilled and qualified. To this end, National Occupational Standards (NOS) have been developed by SkillsActive and approved by the Qualifications and Curriculum Authority (QCA). These standards help define job roles and offer descriptions of skills and knowledge required to perform various roles within the industry. Qualifications in the industry are closely aligned with the NOS so that individuals who hold specific qualifications will have demonstrated the NOS skills specific to their qualification.

THE REGISTER OF EXERCISE PROFESSIONALS (REPS)

In many industries there is a requirement for a professional body membership before an individual can practise. Currently in the health and fitness industry there is no requirement for membership to practise, however, the Register of Exercise Professionals (REPs) has been set up to help safeguard and to promote the health and interests of people who are using the services of exercise and fitness instructors, teachers and trainers. Most employers are now looking for membership of REPs in their potential employees. REPs uses a process of self-regulation that recognises industry-based qualifications, practical competency, and requires fitness professionals to work to a Code of Ethical Practice (see appendix 1) within the framework of National Occupational Standards. In other words, any individual who is accepted onto the Register of Exercise Professionals will have demonstrated appropriate competency relevant to the level to which they have been accepted (this is determined by REPs). Qualifications needed to gain acceptance onto the register are closely aligned with National Occupation Standards for health and fitness as the NOS underpin each of the register's entry categories.

NATIONAL OCCUPATION STANDARDS

These standards are essentially a list of knowledge and skill-based criteria related to areas of health and fitness with progressive levels of competency from level 2 to level 4 (level 1 is simply a registration level and requires no level of competency). Achievement of qualifications at all levels allows entry onto the exercise register.

Table 1.1	NOS Level 2 mandatory and optional units

Level 2 Mandatory unit codes and description

A355	Reflect on and develop own practice in providing exercise and physical activity.
C22	Promote health safety and welfare in active leisure and recreation.
C316	Work with clients to help them to adhere to exercise and physical activity.
	Core knowledge

Level 2 Optional unit codes and description

Gym	D451 – Plan and prepare a gym-based exercise. D452 – Instruct and supervise gym-based exercise.
Exercise to Music	D453 – Plan and prepare group exercise to music. D454 – Instruct group exercise to music.
Aqua	D455 – Plan and prepare water-based exercise. D456 – Instruct water-based exercise.
Physical activity for children	D457 – Plan health related exercise and physical activity for children. D458 – Instruct children in health related exercise and physical activity.

Table 1.2 NOS Level 3 units

Level 3 Area	Unit code and description
Personal trainer	D-460 Design, manage and adapt a personal training programme with clients. D-461 Deliver exercise and physical activity as part of a personal training programme. D-462 Apply the principles of nutrition to support client goals as part of an exercise and physical activity programme.
Exercise referral	D-463 Design, manage and adapt a physical activity programme with referred patients. D-464 Instruct exercise and physical activity with referred patients.
Advanced exercise to music	D-470 Design, manage and adapt an exercise to music programme incorporating advanced teaching strategies. D-471 Deliver exercise to music sessions incorporating advanced teaching strategies.
EMDP/Yoga/Pilates	D-465 Design, manage and adapt a mat EMDP/Yoga/Pilates programme. D-466 Instruct mat Pilates sessions.
All areas	Core knowledge

LEVEL 2: INSTRUCTING EXERCISE AND FITNESS

There are four categories from which to gain entry to Level 2 of the register: gym, exercise to music (ETM), aqua and physical activity for children. Instructors may hold one or more of these categories. In order to gain an award at this level, individuals must successfully complete all of the mandatory units and one or more of the optional units (table 1.1). Individuals must also demonstrate competence of core exercise and fitness knowledge.

Trainers who hold qualifications at level 2 are often employed within private health clubs or public sports and fitness centres. Duties mainly include inductions of set programmes for gym-based individuals or the delivery of group ETM or Aqua sessions.

LEVEL 3: INSTRUCTING PHYSICAL ACTIVITY

There are four categories at Level 3 of the exercise register: fitness instructor/personal trainer, advanced exercise to music, exercise referral and EMDP (exercise, music and dance partnership)/yoga/Pilates. In order to gain a qualification at this level, individuals must successfully complete all of the units related to one or more of the areas as shown in Table 1.2. Individuals must also demonstrate competence of the core exercise and fitness knowledge required at this level. Instructors at this level can choose to remain in employment and carry out more advanced duties such as designing programmes for special populations or they can choose to become self-employed and deliver client-based sessions, either within health and fitness facilities or as a home-based operator.

Table 1.3 Additional register categories

Additional Categories (accessed from either level 2 or 3)

Unit code	Unit description
Older adults	D-467 Adapt a physical activity programme to the needs of older adults.
Disability	D-468 Adapt a physical activity programme to the needs of disabled clients.
Ante/post-natal	D-469 Adapt a physical activity programme to the needs of ante- and postnatal clients.

Those who hold the exercise referral qualification may also work within GP referral schemes, either as an employee or on a consultancy basis.

Having gained a Level 2 or Level 3 award there are additional categories that can be accessed as shown in table 1.3.

Essentially, level 2 and 3 instructors are only qualified to work on a one-to-one or group basis with apparently healthy individuals (unless they hold a relevant qualification for any other population) for whom screening has been carried out (see chapter 3), however, they may on occasion allow appropriately screened and asymptomatic* special population** individuals to take part in mainstream studio, aqua or gym exercise sessions. Trainers must be aware however that if this becomes regular then they must endeavour to become qualified in the appropriate area.

---

* Asymptomatic is the term used to denote the absence of any specified key symptoms of disease identified in screening.

** Special population clients are those deemed by Skills Active to include the following:
- 14–16 year old people
- Disabled people
- Older people (50+)
- Ante- and postnatal women

LEVEL 4: SPECIALIST TRAINER

There are several categories (referred to as medical categories as they are related to clinical environments) at level 4 which trainers can only attempt if they hold a level 3 qualification in exercise referral and a specified number of hours of professional practice. The specialist areas are:

- Cardiac disease
- Falls prevention
- Stroke
- Mental health
- Back pain
- Obesity/diabetes
- Chronic respiratory disease
- Cancer rehabilitation
- Long term neurological conditions
- Military rehab

There is also the intention to have a 'non-medical' category of 'strength and conditioning', which instructors can access, however, for this category the assessment can only be carried out by the UK Strength and Conditioning Society (www.ukscs.org.uk). Employment routes for level 4 qualified trainers are more diverse than those trainers at levels 2 or 3. There are opportunities to work in more clinical environments such as NHS Cardiac Rehab Phase IV centres or stroke rehabilitation units or for local authority health schemes in areas such as mental health and obesity.

CONTINUING PROFESSIONAL DEVELOPMENT (CPD)

Once accepted onto the register, it is the responsibility of trainers to continue their personal development. This can include further qualifications or attending workshops, seminars or conferences, which have been accredited by REPs, in order to remain on the register (trainers can also get points for non-accredited training but it usually means there are fewer allocated points). This is known as 'continuing professional development' or CPD, and members have to undertake a minimum amount of hours in order to stay on the register. It is important that trainers regularly take stock of their performance (see part 1) and update their knowledge base in order to identify any training needs so that they can provide the best possible advice and motivation for clients. This can be done by way of appraisal with other industry professionals with a view to developing a personal action plan with regards to the identification of CPD training.

Did you know?

Trainers on the register must have current public liability insurance and they must ensure that their insurance covers all the populations that they are qualified to instruct.

ROLE OF THE INSTRUCTOR

The main role of the fitness professional is to help change people's lifestyles by way of diet and exercise. It is widely recognised that poor diet and inactivity can affect the risk of developing disease such as coronary heart disease, hypertension, stroke, obesity, diabetes, cancers and many other conditions yet despite the well-documented health benefits of a physically active lifestyle, much of the adult population remains sedentary. For this reason the government has highlighted in many of its 'Health of a Nation' documents the need for a change in people's diet and exercise habits.

Research has generally shown that new clients often exude high levels of motivation when first starting a programme of exercise and are subsequently willing to adopt new exercise behaviours with little encouragement from the trainer. However there are also clients who will need a great deal of encouragement and regular reinforcement from the trainer. Essentially, most clients will fit into one of two categories; those with existing medical conditions for whom a lifestyle change will help to improve or at least prevent decline of the condition and those apparently healthy for whom a lifestyle change will help to prevent or reduce the risk of future conditions. Regardless of the type of client it is the responsibility of the instructor to work within guidelines known as the 'Code of Ethical Practice'.

CODE OF ETHICAL PRACTICE

The Code of Ethical Practice in the health and fitness industry outlines good practice in four main areas: rights, relationships, responsibilities and standards (see appendix 1). When joining the Register of Exercise Professionals, trainers assent to abide by this code and in turn accept their responsibility to themselves; to people who participate in exercise; to other fitness professionals and colleagues; to their respective fitness associations, professional bodies and institutes; to their employer; and to society.

In the unfortunate event of a client complaint, the trainer should always remain professional in the way in which they deal with it. A scheduled meeting with the client and another unbiased professional colleague can often be enough to resolve minor complaints (but however small make sure they are recorded in note form or audio format and a copy given to all parties). In more serious cases of alleged professional misconduct or failure to comply with the terms of membership of the register, clients making the complaint can be referred to the Professional Practice Committee of the Fitness Alliance, which will consider any need for sanctions. Guidance from the committee could also be sought in cases where disagreement or conflict between colleagues cannot be resolved. However, every effort should be made in the first instance to do so using the Code of Ethical Practice as a template to base any resolution on.

It is recommended that trainers always make potential clients aware of their rights to make a complaint. This should be done as early as possible, either by talking them through the process, or showing them the appropriate literature. As a programme of regular exercise has been shown to contribute positively to the physiological, psychological and emotional development of individuals, it is important that trainers are aware of and abide fully by this code. As a guide to abiding by the code of ethics the trainer should consider the following areas:

POSITIVE IMAGE

It's thought that an opinion will be formed in the first few seconds of meeting someone for the first time, which means first impressions are vital. The trainer should act in a professional manner at all times, so when meeting someone for the first time it's worthwhile to keep the acronym PEAP in mind:

P – Polite: shake hands and state your name
E – Eye contact: maintain eye contact at all times
A – Appearance: be professional in your appearance and set an example
P – Person's name: listen carefully and remember the name of the person

TRAINER–CLIENT RELATIONSHIP

According to research (Griffin, 2006), if the trainer successfully establishes a relationship of trust with their client, the client is more likely to stick to the exercise programme. Griffin states that the client's willingness to engage is largely dependent on the inter-personal skills of the trainer, and so this skill should be constantly developed. Griffin suggests that this can be developed by asking 'open-ended' questions (which are those that allow the client to expand on a point rather than giving a yes or no answer) or closed questions (yes or no response) when appropriate. It's also important to show empathy to clients such as by saying (truthfully!) 'I completely understand as I have been through that myself', which will help gain the client's trust. These and other skills such as communication, listening and giving feedback are covered later in this book.

DEFINING BOUNDARIES

At the start of any client relationship it's important that the trainer makes the client fully aware of exactly what they can offer so that clients cannot be mislead in any way when agreeing to take on their services. The trainer should let the client know that should a service be needed that is outside the range of the trainer's skills, they may refer them to another health professional. This will be discussed further throughout the book.

VALUING THE CLIENT

One of the clear messages within the Code of Ethical Practice relates to valuing all clients equally (referred to as valuing diversity) regardless of their class, gender, sexuality, culture, religion or race. It is important that instructors value all clients equally and adapt their service to the specific needs of each client as far as it is practically possible in order to avoid potential discrimination that clients might experience. For example, there are certain religions such as Islam where it is considered inappropriate for females to exercise, therefore, if the trainer is faced with this situation, the exercise sessions may be done behind closed doors and with a female trainer.

MAINTAIN CONFIDENTIALITY

There are many issues relating to the term 'confidentiality' which will be explored in detail. In simple terms, confidentiality relates to keeping any information that is passed between two persons (trainer–client or trainer–colleague) confidential and not shared with others without permission. As long as trainers adhere to the Code of Ethical Practice and guidelines given within this book, confidentiality will not be a cause for concern.

REFLECTIVE PRACTICE AND PROFESSIONAL DEVELOPMENT

2

THE NOS LEVEL 3 PERSONAL TRAINER CRITERIA COVERED IN THIS CHAPTER ARE:

- The aspects of your professional practice that you should reflect upon
- Information that you should use
- Different methods of collecting information and how to interpret it
- How to reflect on your own practice
- How to identify key lessons and how to make use of these in the future
- The importance of discussing your ideas with another professional
- How often you should review your professional practice
- How to access information on developments in exercise and physical activity
- How to identify areas in which you need to develop your professional practice further
- The importance of having a personal action plan for your development
- The types of development activities that are available to you and how to access these
- The importance of regularly reviewing and updating your personal action plan
- Why continuous improvement is important for physical activity instructors
- Why it is important to prioritise the improvement of some programme components
- How to prioritise which programme components to work on
- Sources of information, advice and best practice on how to improve programme components
- Why it is important to share your conclusions about improving your own practice with other people
- Who you can share your ideas for improvement with
- How to make use of improvements in the future

REFLECTIVE PRACTICE

Reflective practice is defined by Gillie Bolton (2010) as 'an in-depth consideration of events or situations, the people involved, what they experienced, and how they felt about it'. A trainer who uses this practice in order to improve his or her service will try to identify what did not go as expected during sessions – good or bad – and the possible reasons why the session went the way it did. Reflective thinking also takes into account the views of others, including those of clients and colleagues. As effective reflection can be relatively time-consuming it is recommended that it is done regularly but not so often as to reduce the effectiveness of the process. There are many reasons for instructors to use reflective practice including:

- Helps to keep up to date with developments in exercise and physical activity
- Helps to consider and focus on career goals and aspirations
- Identifies areas needed to develop professional practice further

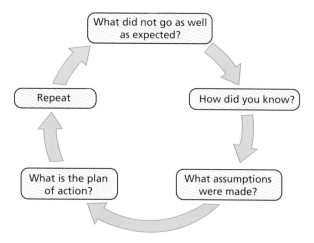

Figure 2.1 A typical cyclical reflection model

- Helps to develop a personal action plan to improve professional practice

There are many different types of reflective models, however, the cyclical reflection model (see figure 2.1) is a simple and effective one for instructors to use to help improve their service.

The process can best be described by using a typical example related to the delivery of a training session within the health and fitness environment:

Example: A cardio session that was performed by a regular client.

- *What did not go as well as expected?* – The client seemed lethargic and unmotivated.
- *How did you know?* – The client might have been asked to complete an evaluation of the session in which they stated that they felt slightly under the weather.
- *What assumptions were made?* – The instructor may have assumed that as the client enjoyed previous sessions that they would have enjoyed this one too. Assumptions could also have been made that a visual screening of the client showed no indication of illness.
- *What is the plan of action?* – In this particular case the instructor could implement a more rigorous pre-session screening process and try to elicit more regular feedback from the client during the session.
- *Repeat* – The session would then be repeated on another occasion taking into account the actions and the process would repeat itself.

INTRODUCTORY SESSION ASSESSMENT FORM

	Client: Date:	A = Colleague B = Instructor	A	B
Collect and record information about clients				
1	Establish a rapport with clients		✓	✗
2	Explain your role and responsibilities to the clients		✗	✓
3	Decide what information you need to collect about clients		✓	✓
4	Collect information about clients using appropriate methods		✓	✓
5	Show sensitivity and empathy to clients and the information they provide		✓	✓
6	Record the information in a way that will help you analyse it		✓	✓
7	Identify when clients need referral to another professional		✓	✓
8	Treat confidential information correctly		✓	✓
Analyse information and agree goals with clients				
9	Analyse the information you collected		✓	✓
10	Identify any barriers to participation and encourage clients to find a solution		✓	✓
11	Agree with clients their needs and readiness to participate		✓	✓
12	Work with clients to agree short, medium and long-term goals appropriate to their needs		✓	✓
13	Make sure the goals are specific, measurable, achievable, realistic and time bound and reflect accepted good practice		✓	✓
14	Record the agreed goals in a format that is clear to clients, yourself and others who may be involved in the programme		✗	✓
15	Identify and agree strategies to prevent drop out or relapse		✓	✓

Difference criteria numbers = 1, 2, 14

Plan of action strategies:
1. No action to be taken as discussion with colleague highlighted there appeared to be a good rapport with client.
2. Didn't outline responsibilities. Could provide client with Code of Ethics.
3. Colleague informed that client seemed vague in response to understanding the goals. Improve communication and develop alternative recording format.

Figure 2.2 Introductory session assessment form. (For a template visit: www.bloomsbury.com/9781408187234)

The reason that the model is cyclical in nature is that repeating sessions (taking into account the plan of action) might not resolve the initial issue, therefore, the trainer would need to assess the repeat session to identify if the issue had been resolved or a new issue identified. As the process of effective reflection can often be unfamiliar to the trainer, the use of specific assessment tools, such as those identified in figures 2.2 to 2.5, can help to improve delivery of the service during both the client introductory, on-going and review sessions (as covered later in this book) by focusing on particular areas of delivery such as:

- how effective the physical activities were
- how effective and motivational the relationship was with the client
- how well professional codes of ethics were implemented
- how well the instructing style matched each client's needs
- how well the client's exercise was managed, including their health, safety and welfare
- how good interaction and working with other members of staff was

SESSION PLANNING ASSESSMENT FORM

Client: Date: A = Colleague B = Instructor   A   B

Plan and prepare individualised exercise sessions

		A	B
1	Provide a range of exercises to help clients achieve their objectives and goals	✓	✓
2	Select teaching styles that are appropriate to the exercises and clients	✓	✓
3	Plan and agree the focus of exercises and utilise the resources available, improvising safely where necessary	✓	✓
4	Plan realistic timings, intensities and sequences of exercises	✗	✓
5	Make sure there is an effective balance of instruction, activity and discussion within the session	✓	✓
6	Identify, obtain and prepare the resources you need for the planned exercises	✓	✓

Difference criteria numbers = 4

Plan of action strategies:
1. Colleague identified that starting intensity may be too high for client based on background history. Confirm this with appropriate text on client condition.

Figure 2.3 Session planning assessment form. (For a template visit: www.bloomsbury.com/9781408187234)

SESSION DELIVERY ASSESSMENT FORM

Client: Date: A = Colleague B = Instructor   A   B

Prepare and teach an individualised exercise session

		A	B
1	Meet clients punctually and make them feel at ease	✓	✓
2	Collect any new information from clients about response to previous activity	✓	✓
3	Discuss the objectives and exercises that you have planned for the session and how these link to clients' goals	✓	✓
4	Discuss the physical and technical demands of the planned exercises and how clients can progress or regress these to meet their goals	✗	✓
5	Assess, agree and review clients' state of readiness and motivation to take part in the planned exercises	✓	✓
6	Negotiate, agree and record with clients any changes to the planned exercises that will meet their goals and preferences and enable them to maintain progress	✓	✓

Teach and adapt planned exercises

		A	B
7	Use teaching and motivational styles that are appropriate to clients and accepted good practice	✓	✓
8	Provide clients with an appropriate warm-up	✓	✓
9	Make best use of the environment in which clients are exercising	✓	✓
10	Provide instructions, explanations and demonstrations that are technically correct, safe and effective	✓	✓
11	Check clients' understanding of instructions, explanations and demonstrations	✓	✓
12	Adapt verbal and non-verbal communication methods to make sure clients understand what is required	✗	✓
13	Ensure clients can carry out the exercises safely on their own	✓	✓
14	Observe and analyse clients' performance, providing positive reinforcement throughout	✓	✓
15	Correct techniques at appropriate points	✓	✓

| 16 | Progress or regress exercises according to clients' performance | ✓ | ✓ |

Bring exercise sessions to an end

17	Allow sufficient time for the closing phase of the session	✓	✓
18	End the exercises using a cool down that is safe and effective for clients	✓	✓
19	Provide clients with positive reinforcement about their performance	✗	✓
20	Give clients your feedback on the session	✓	✓
21	Explain to clients how their progress links to short-, medium- and long-term goals	✓	✓
22	Discuss other possible activities with your clients	✓	✓
23	Leave the environment in a condition suitable for future use	✓	✓

Difference criteria numbers = 4, 12, 19

Plan of action strategies:
1. Forgot to discuss demands of exercise session. Use a checklist in future.
2. Could have used non-verbal cues at times to reinforce technique. Try to do this in next session for all exercises.
3. Negative feedback needs to be given with positive. Try the sandwich method.

Figure 2.4 Session delivery assessment form. (For a template visit: www.bloomsbury.com/9781408187234)

The assessment forms have been adapted from National Occupational Standards so that the views of others are taken into consideration. This requires a more experienced colleague to observe particular sessions, so the permission of the client would need to be sought before the session is observed. The colleague should be made aware of the assessment form used prior to the session so that they are familiar with the process. During the observed session the colleague should indicate with a tick in column A if, in their opinion, each criteria was met effectively. At the end of the session the instructor could do the same by judging their own performance. Any difference in opinion could be identified at the foot of the assessment form which could then be discussed between the colleague and instructor, this is essentially the 'how did you know?' stage of the cyclical reflection model. Taking into account the views of the colleague, the trainer could then devise appropriate strategies ('what is the plan of action?' stage) in order to address the issues that were discussed previously. The views of the client can also be taken into consideration using the same assessment forms. However, the forms may have to be amended to suit the client or explained fully

PERSONAL TRAINING

		Date:	A = Colleague B = Instructor	A	B
Client:					

Review progress with clients

		A	B
1	Monitor clients' progress using appropriate methods	✓	✓
2	Review progress with clients at agreed points in the programme	✓	✓
3	Make sure clients understand the purpose of review and how it fits into their programme	✓	✓
4	Encourage clients to give their own views on progress	✓	✓
5	Use agreed evaluation guidelines	✗	✓
6	Give positive and timely feedback to clients during their review	✓	✓
7	Agree review outcomes with clients and keep an accurate record	✓	✓

Adapt a personal training programme with clients

		A	B
8	Identify goals and activities that need to be redefined or adapted	✓	✓
9	Agree adaptations, progressions or regressions to meet clients' needs as and when necessary to optimise their achievement	✗	✓
10	Identify and agree any changes to resources and environments	✓	✓
11	Introduce adaptations in a way that is appropriate to clients and their needs	✓	✓
12	Record changes to your plans for the programme to take account of adaptations	✓	✓
13	Monitor the effectiveness of your adaptations and update these as necessary	✓	✓

Difference criteria numbers = 5, 9

Plan of action strategies:
1. Progression not linked back to original client goals. Consider this for next review.
2. Didn't consider recommended clinical guidelines in terms of adaptation alternatives. Develop more understanding of the client condition.

Figure 2.5 Review session assessment form. (For a template visit: www.bloomsbury.com/9781408187234)

prior to use. The views of the client can also be taken into consideration using the Service Quality Questionnaire, which is discussed later in the book in chapter 17.

PERSONAL DEVELOPMENT

Reflective practice provides an ideal opportunity for self-development, however, it is important that the instructor uses the various session assessment forms systematically. Looking over these forms can help to identify any specific areas that the trainer might wish to develop with training. One method to help do this is to synthesise and review information using a Personal Development Action Plan (PDAP) as shown in figure 2.6 overleaf.

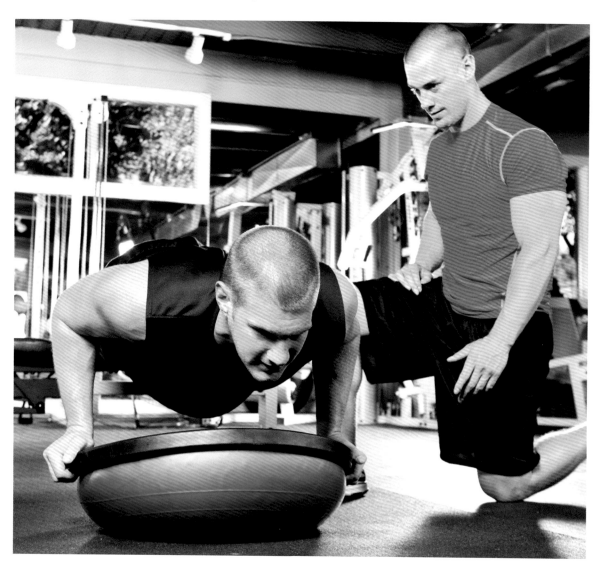

Date of assessed session:

REFLECTION STRATEGIES	NEEDS	✓
Introduction session strategies:		
1 No action to be taken as discussion with colleague highlighted there appeared to be a good rapport with client.	N/A	
2 Didn't outline responsibilities. Could provide client with Code of Ethics.	Code of Ethics needed for next session.	
3 Colleague informed that client seemed vague in response to understanding the goals. Improve communication and develop alternative recording format.	Investigate alternative recording formats.	
Planning strategies:		
1 Colleague identified that starting intensity may be too high for client based on background history. Confirm this with appropriate text on client condition.	Check appropriate intensities prior to next session.	
Delivery strategies:		
1 Forgot to discuss demands of exercise session. Use a checklist in future.	Produce checklist prior to next session.	
2 Could have used non-verbal cues at times to reinforce technique. Try to do this in next session for all exercises.	Mental reminder for start of next session.	
3 Negative feedback needs to be given with positive. Try the sandwich method.	Read appropriate text on sandwich feedback method.	
Review strategies:		
1 Progression not linked back to original client goals. Consider this for next review.	Review and consider training course.	
2 Didn't consider recommended clinical guidelines in terms of adaptation alternatives. Develop more understanding of the client condition.	Read appropriate text and consider training course.	

PERSONAL TRAINING

Training requirement:

1 – Goal setting

2 – Specific course related to client condition.

Potential training provider:

Figure 2.6 Personal Development Action Plan. (For a template visit: www.bloomsbury.com/9781408187234)

There are many reasons why it is important to involve more experienced people in reflective practice. Their objective viewpoints can help to identify areas of the exercise programme that could be improved, how to prioritise these areas and how best to develop action plans to address the improvement. It is important to link a time-frame to these needs so that during the next reflective practice they can be marked as complete or on-going to make it easier to track. The PDAP also allows for recording any specific training requirement and potential training provider necessary. It is important that instructors regularly review and update PDAPs as they can help to identify areas of development that might be needed.

To help instructors develop their skills, Skills-Active provide information on their website relating to all accredited continuing professional development (CPD) courses, workshops, seminars, events, etc., ranging from those suitable for level 2 trainers to those suitable for level 4 trainers.

PART TWO
PLAN EXERCISE PROGRAMMES

COLLECT AND REVIEW CLIENT INFORMATION

3

THE NOS LEVEL 3 PERSONAL TRAINER CRITERIA COVERED IN THIS CHAPTER ARE:

- Why it is important to collect accurate information about your clients
- How to decide what information to collect
- Safe and appropriate methods you can use to collect the information you need
- Formats for recording information
- The legal and ethical implications of collecting information about clients
- Why it is important to work together with clients to agree goals and activities
- The importance of long-term behaviour change and how to ensure clients understand and commit themselves to long-term change
- Behavioural psychology and different approaches to behaviour change
- The importance of being sensitive to clients' goals and current stage of readiness
- How to organise information in a way which will help to interpret and analyse it
- How to analyse and interpret collected information to identify clients' needs and goals
- The importance of clients understanding the advantages of taking part in a personal training programme and identifying any obstacles they may face
- Why it is important to base goal setting on analysis of clients' needs
- Barriers which may prevent clients achieving their goals
- Why it is important to identify and agree short-, medium- and long-term goals with clients and ensure that these take account of barriers and discrepancies, including client fears and reservations about physical activity
- When to involve others, apart from clients, in goal-setting
- How to develop, agree and record goals which are appropriate to clients
- How to make goals specific, measurable, achievable, realistic and time bound
- Strategies which can prevent drop out or relapse

- How to administer and interpret the Physical Activity Readiness Questionnaire
- The types of medical conditions that will prevent you from working with a client unless you have specialist training and qualifications
- When you should refer clients to other professionals and the procedures to follow
- The importance of safeguarding confidentiality of collected information and how to do so
- The strengths and weaknesses of the various methods of collecting information for different types of clients
- How to make sure you have the informed consent of clients before collecting information
- Legal and organisational requirements for data protection and confidentiality
- Why thorough planning and preparation are necessary
- How to include physical activities as part of each client's lifestyle
- Different strategies to enable clients to change their behaviour and achieve their goals
- The typical goals and expectations that clients have
- The types of barriers individual clients may face when undertaking physical activity and achieving their goals
- How you can help clients overcome these barriers
- The types of incentives and rewards appropriate to a range of different clients
- The types of exercise preferences that different clients may have
- How to assist clients to develop their own adherence strategies

THE 6-STEP CLIENT PATHWAY

When trainers take on a new client it is important that they follow the same procedures each time in order to design an exercise programme targeted to the client's needs. To help trainers a standardised system known as The 6-Step Client Pathway should be used (see figure 3.1). This system organises your clients' information in a way that it can be easily analysed, interpreted and stored for future access. It's important to ensure that information relating to clients is dealt with in line with the Data Protection Act 1998. Essentially, the Data Protection Act determines your responsibilities when collecting and keeping information. The main areas are:

- Personal data should only be collected for lawful purposes

- Personal data should only be used for the purposes for which it has been collected
- Personal data should not be kept for longer than is necessary
- Measures should be taken to ensure that personal data is kept confidential and stored appropriately

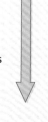

1. Screening
2. Identify stage of change
3. Agree goals
4. Identify health and fitness components
5. Test components
6. Programme design

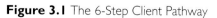

Figure 3.1 The 6-Step Client Pathway

Following the 6-Step Client Pathway helps the trainer to identify and overcome any physical or mental barriers that the client may have, and establish goals to work towards, leading to a greater chance of success.

The first session with a new client should focus on gathering information that enables the trainer to design an exercise programme targeted specifically for that client. The trainer should make sure the client is aware of this process and consents to it. The trainer should assure the client that the information they give you is confidential and will be treated in accordance with the Data Protection Act of 1998. Trainers may find it helpful to provide their clients with a written copy of the act, which is available online at www.legislation.gov.uk/ukpga/1998/29/contents.

SCREENING

The trainer should first screen the client for any health issues and, if necessary, refer them to the appropriate colleague or health professional before they undertake an exercise programme. Always ask the client's permission before any referral takes place. Explain to the client that they will be unable to exercise until the referral has taken place, and after any issues are resolved.

BEHAVIOUR CHANGE

The trainer should then establish how motivated the client is to change their behaviour (see page 27). This will help identify the strategy the PT uses as part of the programme design.

GOALS

The client's goals should always be discussed. Are they performance related, looking to improve their health or just wanting to have fun?

It's importance to link any fitness strategy or programme to these goals.

NEEDS ANALYSIS

Once the goals of the client have been identified and agreed with the trainer, each component of health/fitness that is necessary to achieve the goals should be identified. This is sometimes called a 'needs analysis'. For example: does the client want to build up their cardiovascular endurance? Does this involve running at a constant or varied pace?

TESTING

At this stage, the client should be tested to identify a baseline level from which a programme can be developed. Each component must be put into a comprehensive training plan (normally a minimum period of one year but depends on the goals) that shows when and which components will be developed and when follow-up testing of these components would take place.

SCREENING

The main purpose of screening is to help individuals determine their current health and fitness status before undertaking a programme of exercise. Not only can this aid in planning and designing a safe and effective programme, it can also help in identifying any health issues that may need advice from a health professional, such as a doctor or physiotherapist.

In the health and fitness industry there are two methods of screening commonly used: pre-exercise questionnaires and verbal screening.

PRE-EXERCISE QUESTIONNAIRES

Many types of pre-exercise health questionnaires are available to the trainer; the most common being the Physical Activity Readiness Questionnaire, or PAR-Q (see figure 3.2). Originally developed by the Canadian Society for Exercise Physiology, the PAR-Q is a short questionnaire that can help to identify possible symptoms of cardiovascular, pulmonary and metabolic disease, as well as other conditions that might be aggravated by exercise. If any conditions are identified, the form advises the individual to seek medical approval (see page 28) prior to undertaking a programme of exercise, unless the trainer holds a specific qualification related to the identified condition and feels fully confident to deal with it. These conditions include: coronary heart disease; respiratory conditions; type 2 diabetes; bone and joint problems; and mental health. During the screening process the trainer should ask the client if they have any conditions that they think might be important in relation to exercise. If no conditions are identified, the form suggests a programme of light to moderate exercise. It is advised that PAR-Q forms should be completed in full by the client before any other information is gathered. If the trainer feels that the form reveals anything that is beyond their training or experience, they should refer the case to a suitably qualified colleague or health professional. It should also be noted that PAR-Qs are normally only valid for a 12-month period.

The PAR-Q screening process can also help to identify certain conditions that have been shown to increase the risk of heart disease, known as coronary artery disease risk factors. This process is known as 'risk stratification'. On completion of a risk stratification questionnaire, such as that in figure 3.3, individuals are classified into one of three categories: low risk (or apparently healthy), moderate risk or high risk (refer to ACSM (2009) for more information relating to this process).

Some of the information requested requires specialist testing to have already taken place. If the client has a condition, they should be aware of the results of their tests, as their health is one of the reasons they have been told to undertake a programme of exercise.

The ACSM states that individuals who are in the moderate category should not be prescribed any vigorous exercise unless medical approval is given and individuals in the high-risk category should not be allowed to exercise unless supervised by a qualified person, following medical approval. If in any doubt, the trainer should refer the client to a health professional, such as their GP, before any programme of exercise. In some cases, and with the client's consent, the trainer may collaborate with other professionals when designing the exercise programme.

VERBAL SCREENING

In addition to the PAR-Q screening form, trainers should screen clients verbally prior to an exercise session. There may have been a period of time between a client completing a PAR-Q and beginning a programme of exercise during which injuries may have occurred, so clients should always be asked if they know of any reason why they should not exercise or if they have any current injury that could prevent them from exercising. It is at the trainer's discretion to decide whether any response warrants medical referral. Verbal screening is also confidential, therefore, discretion must be used in a group exercise situation.

IDENTIFY STAGE OF CHANGE

Starting an exercise programme often requires a change in lifestyle and habits on the part of the individual. This is commonly known as 'behavioural

Please read the following questions and answer each one honestly.   Yes   No

1   Has your doctor ever said that you have a heart condition and that you should only do physical activity recommended by a doctor?

2   Do you feel pain in your chest when you do physical activity?

3   In the past month, have you had chest pain while you were not doing physical activity?

4   Do you lose your balance because of dizziness or do you ever lose consciousness?

5   Do you have a bone or joint problem that could be made worse by physical activity?

6   Is your doctor currently prescribing drugs for your blood pressure or heart condition?

7   Do you know of any other reason why you should not do physical activity?

If you answered YES to one or more questions:
Talk to your doctor BEFORE you become more physically active or have a fitness appraisal. Discuss with your doctor which kinds of activities you wish to participate in.

If you answered NO to all questions you can be reasonably sure that you can:
• Start becoming much more physically active. Start slowly and build up gradually.
• Take part in a fitness appraisal. This is a good way to determine your basic fitness level. It is recommended that you have your blood pressure evaluated.
However, delay becoming active if:
• You are not feeling well because of temporary illness such as a cold or 'flu.
• You are or may be pregnant: talk to your doctor first.

Please note: If your health changes so that you then answer YES to any of the above questions, tell your fitness or health professional. Ask whether you should change your physical activity plan.

'I have read, understood and completed this questionnaire. Any questions I had were answered to my full satisfaction.'

Name: Signature of witness:

Signature: Signature of parent/guardian:

Date: Note: This physical activity clearance is valid for a maximum of 12 months from the date it is completed, and becomes invalid if your condition changes so that you would answer YES to any of the seven questions.

Figure 3.2 Example of Physical Activity Readiness Questionnaire (Source: Physical Activity Readiness Questionnaire (PAR-Q) 2002. Reprinted with permission from the Canadian Society for Exercise Physiology.) (for a blank template please visit: www.bloomsbury.com/9781408187234).

change'. Unfortunately, many people change their habits in the short-term but do not persist with the change long enough for it to become a new behaviour. Research has suggested that behavioural change is a long-term process, and it can be challenging for both the client and the trainer to overcome habits that have been in place for many years. However, models such as Prochaska and DiClemente's 'Stages of Change' model can help trainers to facilitate the process.

RISK STRATIFICATION QUESTIONNAIRE

Client name:

D.O.B.   Date

Please answer the following questions to the best of your knowledge: Yes   No

1   Has there been a heart attack or sudden death before age 55 (father, brother or son) or before age 65 (mother, sister or daughter) in your family?

2   Are you a current smoker or quit within previous six months?

3   Have you been diagnosed with systolic blood pressure 140mmhg or above, or diastolic of 90mmhg or above, on at least two occasions?

4   Do you have total serum cholesterol of more than 5.2mmol/L, or LDL more than 3.4mmol/L, or HDL less than 1.03mmol/L?

5   Is your BMI $30kg/m^2$ or above?

6   Are you sedentary?

7   Is your impaired fasting glucose: 100mg/dL or more?

Sub-total number of 'Yes' answers:

Is your HDL level above 1.6mmol/L. If yes, subtract 1 from the total above.

Total number of 'Yes' answers:

Low risk	**Moderate risk**	**High risk**
Men ≥45: women ≥55 and no more than 1 'Yes' answers	Men ≥45: women ≥55 OR 2 or more 'Yes' answers	Those with known cardiovascular, pulmonary or metabolic disease

Figure 3.3 Adapted risk stratification questionnaire (for a template visit: www.bloomsbury.com/9781408187234).

STAGES OF CHANGE MODEL

Prochaska originally started work on the behavioural change model after his father died of alcoholism and depression. It was in 1982 during collaboration with DiClemente that they identified common phases that smokers went through to change their behaviour and subsequently proposed the Stages of Change model, which proposes that there are a number of stages of readiness related to change. Over the years the model has been adapted, often by psychologists, to help clients stop smoking, relieve dependency on alcohol and help with exercise uptake.

In order to identify which stage of change a client might be at, trainers can use the Stages of Change questionnaire (as shown in figure 3.5). On completion of the questionnaire by the client, the trainer should use the scoring system to identify which stage they are at.

Clients can relapse at any stage of the process and move back and forth between stages (known as a cyclical process) without progressing to the end stage. Research, such as that by Stone and Klein in 2004, has shown that about 50% of exercisers terminate activity within 3–6 months of beginning a training programme. In an attempt to help people cope effectively with situations that might trigger relapse, Marlatt and Gordon (1985) proposed a 'Relapse Prevention Model'. Although originally designed to enhance abstinence of behaviours such as smoking and substance abuse, the model can be applied to exercise and can be summarised as follows:

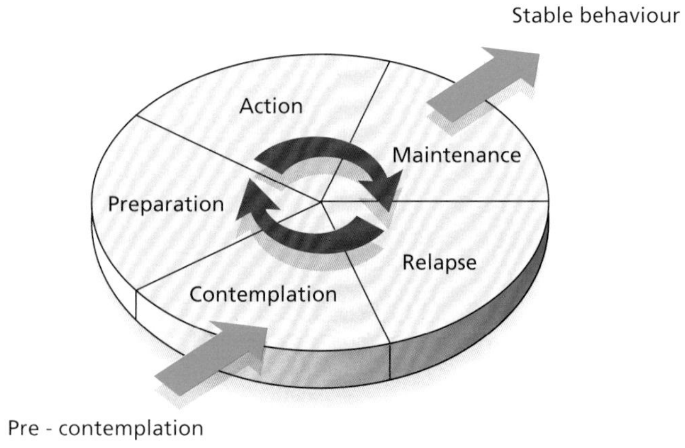

1. Identify typical situations that would trigger relapse (similar to barriers, see page 37).
2. Plan strategies to avoid or cope with triggers (potential solutions, see page 37).
3. De-emphasise the consequences of relapse (e.g. missing a session here and there is not a disaster).
4. Plan for certain lapses (going on holiday, work, etc).
5. Promote intrinsic rewards and the positives of exercise (benefit versus cost, see page 32).

STAGE STRATEGIES

Once the client's stage of change has been identified using the Stages of Change Questionnaire there are strategies that can be employed that can help to move the client to the next stage. Trainers should try to move the client to each progressive stage until they have empowered them to work independently.

Research has shown that matching the strategy to the appropriate stage of change has a greater chance of success. Common strategies that can be used are detailed in table 3.1 and can be noted on the client's goal setting questionnaire (see page 38.).

Whatever strategy the trainer decides to use they should be aware of several fundamental

Figure 3.4 Stages of change processes

STAGES OF CHANGE QUESTIONNAIRE

Physical activity includes activities such as brisk walking, jogging, cycling, swimming, or any other activity, such as gardening, in which the exertion makes you feel warmer or slightly out of breath.

		No	Yes
1	I am currently physically active	0	1
2	I intend to become more physically active in the next 6 months	0	1

For activity to be *regular*, it must add up to a *total* of 30 minutes or more per day and be done at least 5 days per week. For example, you could take one 30-minute walk or take three 10-minute walks.

		No	Yes
3	I currently engage in regular physical activity	0	1
4	I have been regularly physically active for the past 6 months	0	1

Scoring
If (question 1 = 0 and question 2 = 0) then you are at stage 1.
If (question 1 = 0 and question 2 = 1) then you are at stage 2.
If (question 1 = 1 and question 3 = 0) then you are at stage 3.
If (question 1 = 1, question 3 = 1, and question 4 = 0) then you are at stage 4.
If (question 1 = 1, question 3 = 1, and question 4 = 1) then you are at stage 5.

Client name

Date   Stage

Figure 3.5 Adapted Stages of Change Questionnaire (for a template visit: www.bloomsbury.com/9781408187234).

principles relating to the success of exercise adherence that can be used at appropriate stages:

Rewards

During the action and maintenance stages (stages 4 and 5) many trainers use rewards as an incentive for clients. Rewards can include small gifts such as T-shirts, drink bottles, vouchers or cash incentives such as free-sessions. Research, such as that by King in 1992, supports the theory that in the short-term this has a positive effect on exercise adherence. However, according to research, such as that by Glanz and Rimmer in 1995, extrinsic rewards (rewards received from other people) should be replaced in the long term by intrinsic rewards (rewards one finds within oneself, such as enjoyment and self-satisfaction). Programmes based on extrinsic rewards alone do not help people stay active over the long term.

Table 3.1 Identifiers and strategies associated with stages of change

Identifier	Strategy
1. Pre-contemplation • Clients are not considering changing their behaviour • Clients feel that the negatives of changing outweigh the positives	Get clients thinking about change. Show evidence of effects of an unhealthy lifestyle. Promote the benefits of change in terms of health and morbidity.
2. Contemplation • The client is considering change • Negatives don't outweigh positives • Barriers to exercise are now the issue	Reinforcement of health/social messages is key. The trainer should focus on the next stage in helping clients to prepare to take action by regularly re-iterating the benefits of change and the consequences of not changing.
3. Preparation • Clients are serious about changing in the immediate future • Attempts at change may have been made but they have not worked	The main goal is to help clients move to the next stage of taking action. Trainers should develop a plan to change. Goal setting at this stage is important.
4. Action • The client has changed their behaviour within the past 6 months	As this stage is associated with a high risk of relapse, the trainer's priority is to prevent relapse occurring. Try to empower the client by promoting confidence or identify mechanisms of support such as training buddies.
5. Maintenance • The client has maintained the change of behaviour for at least six months	This stage is associated with a decreased risk of relapse but regular re-evaluation of goals and programme can help.
6. Stable behaviour • Clients can now be left to be independent	Empowering a client to be independent is one of the main aims of the trainer.

Visual reminders

Early research, such as that by Brownell in 1980, found that the use of simple visual reminders, such as role-model pictures on fridges, encouraged people to be more active during the action and maintenance stages.

Benefit versus cost

Early research by Janis and Mann in 1997 in the area of decision-making suggested that people are more likely to be active if they believe the benefits of exercise outweigh the costs or disadvantages. It is generally thought that this is more important in the early stages (pre-contemplation and contemplation). Trainers could ask their clients to note down benefits and costs and use appropriate strategies to overcome the perceived costs. For example, the trainer could point out that the cost of a gym membership with its potential long-term health benefits would far outweigh the problems associated with an unhealthy lifestyle.

Joint decisions

Research in the area of behavioural choice, such as that by Epstein in 1998, suggests that if people perceive they are not involved in the process of choosing their behaviour they are less likely to be motivated to change their lifestyle. It is important, therefore, to involve the client in the choices of exercise they make during the preparation stage so that they perceive they are making a contribution to their own programme.

Circumstances

There are many factors in everyday life that promotes sedentary behaviour over physical activity. Behaviour change that relates to these factors is more commonly known as the 'ecological model'. Research in this area, such as that by Badland and Scholfield in 2005, has highlighted that the physical environment can affect exercise participation, especially in the pre-contemplation stage. For example: in the workplace lifts are often more visible than the stairs and it is unsafe to cycle or jog in some areas. Trainers should work with clients to identify these types of barriers and devise strategies (the range of which is beyond the scope of this book) such as encouraging the use of stairs and locating bike trails. It is also useful for the client to enlist the support of friends, family and co-workers by informing them of their life-style change choices as they can often be a source of external motivation which might help to avoid potential relapse.

Promote confidence

Confidence in one's own ability to succeed is also known as 'self-efficacy' and is extremely important in relation to the stages of change. As part of the 'social cognitive theory' proposed by Bandura in the 1980s, it was shown that high levels of self-efficacy expectations lead to positive outcomes, so it is important to set goals that are achievable (see SMART goals) in order to increase self-efficacy and motivation.

Generally speaking, the higher the self-efficacy an individual has, the higher the goals that can be set. Any failure is often attributed to lack of effort and they therefore try harder. On the other hand, individuals with low self-efficacy may attribute failure to low ability, rather than lack of effort, and are more likely to give up. Goal setting on a regular basis (from the preparation stage through to stable behaviour) is of paramount importance especially if self-efficacy is low.

MEASURING SELF-EFFICACY

One of the most common measurement tools is the Self-Efficacy for Exercise (SEE) scale (see figure 3.6) which focuses on how self-efficacious people are, which is related to the ability to continue exercising in the face of barriers to exercise. The SEE consists of situations that might affect a client's current participation in exercise. For each situation, the subject uses the scale from 0 (not confident) to 10 (very confident) to describe their current confidence that they could exercise 3 times a week for 20 minutes each time. As with all client testing, a baseline measurement should be taken prior to the start of the programme to establish the confidence levels of the individual at that particular time. Subsequent tests would then show if confidence had improved, and if so goals could be set or adjusted in relation to this. If a record is kept by the trainer (see PT guide – Goal Setting Questionnaire). it can be used to show that goals were set at the appropriate level for the client's level of confidence at that particular time.

AGREE GOALS

The process of goal setting is a simple, yet often misused motivational technique that can provide some structure for an exercise programme. It is important to do this as it would be unprofessional, and impossible, to design any exercise programme without any specific goals on which to base it. Setting goals can be done in the introductory session with the client. Before agreeing any goals,

SELF-EFFICACY FOR EXERCISE SCALE

How confident are you right now you could exercise 3 times per week for 20 minutes if:	Not Confident	Very Confident
1 You were worried the exercise would cause further pain		0 1 2 3 4 5 6 7 8 9 10
2 You were bored by the programme or activity		0 1 2 3 4 5 6 7 8 9 10
3 You were not sure exactly what exercises to do		0 1 2 3 4 5 6 7 8 9 10
4 You had to exercise alone		0 1 2 3 4 5 6 7 8 9 10
5 You did not enjoy it		0 1 2 3 4 5 6 7 8 9 10
6 You were too busy with other activities		0 1 2 3 4 5 6 7 8 9 10
7 You felt tired during or after exercise		0 1 2 3 4 5 6 7 8 9 10
8 You felt stressed		0 1 2 3 4 5 6 7 8 9 10
9 You felt depressed		0 1 2 3 4 5 6 7 8 9 10
10 You were afraid the exercise would make you fall		0 1 2 3 4 5 6 7 8 9 10
11 You felt pain when exercising		0 1 2 3 4 5 6 7 8 9 10

Client name

Date   Stage of change

Figure 3.6 Adapted Self-Efficacy for Exercise Scale (for a template visit: www.bloomsbury.com/9781408187234).

the trainer should gather as much information as possible about the client's lifestyle of the client so that the goals are specific and achievable.

One of the easiest ways to do this is by using a lifestyle questionnaire. The questionnaire should be as comprehensive as possible but should focus of setting goals, and be tailored to each trainer's expertise and qualifications. A lifestyle questionnaire is not a replacement for the PAR-Q, but rather a supplement to it. There are many lifestyle questionnaires such as the example in figure 3.7.

Goals are usually set in order to accomplish a specific task in a specific period of time, such as losing a certain amount of weight for a wedding or being able to run a half marathon in six months' time. Being specific about the goal helps the individual to focus and direct their activities, and helps to establish a plan of action.

It is important to work together with clients to agree goals and activities as the client can feel as though they have shared ownership of their own programme, which can eventually empower the client to take full ownership when they are ready to do so (Egan, 1990). Clients should also be encouraged to raise any queries or concerns during the assessment, as this helps them to engage in the learning process (Plisk, 2003). However, the trainer should make sure the client knows that,

as goals are based on an analysis of each client's needs, the responsibility of goal setting lies with the trainer, as they have the expertise to set solid and achievable goals.

TYPES OF GOAL

Generally speaking and in relation to exercise, goals can be divided into two distinct types: 'process goals' and 'outcome goals'. as can be seen in table 3.2.

Process goals are where skills are broken down into manageable units that the client can easily focus on. Often form, technique or just participation can be classed as process goals as they are related more to 'just taking part' rather than to results. Outcome goals are concerned with the ultimate outcome, for example, success or failure, winning or losing. In other words, outcome goals are results related as opposed to process goals which are task related. The trainer should be wary of focusing too much on outcome goals as this can mean the process goals are neglected and can result in a poor outcome in terms of injury or reduced performance, especially where the process and outcome goals are linked. Take the example of a client who had a process goal of being able to complete four training sessions a week leading to an outcome goal of completing a half-marathon.

Table 3.2 Examples of process and outcome goals	
Process Goals	**Outcome Goals**
• Be able to join in an aerobics class	• Reduce body fat
• Run or jog without my heart pounding	• Win the county hurdles championship
• Be fit enough to do martial arts every week	• Increase my fitness
• Enjoy the activities I do	• Complete a marathon
	• Reduce a dress size

LIFESTYLE QUESTIONNAIRE

Client name   D.O.B.   Date

Please answer the following questions to the best of your knowledge:

1   Do you currently participate in any form of exercise?

2   How often do you participate in exercise?

3   What types of exercise do you currently participate in?

4   How long do you normally exercise for during each session?

5   Would you class your exercise as moderate or vigorous?

6   Can you walk briskly for 30 minutes without fatigue?

7   Can you jog for 20 minutes without fatigue?

8   What types of exercise do you enjoy doing?

9   What types of exercise do you not like doing?

10   When was the last time you participated in regular exercise?

11   How often and what type of exercise was it?

1   Do you currently smoke and, if so, how much?

2   How much alcohol do you drink on average each week?

3   Do you work at a desk each day?

4   How do you travel to work?

5   What do you do at break times?

6   Are there any stairs at your place of work?

7   What is your typical daily routine?

8   How far do you walk on a typical day

9   Would you consider yourself to have a healthy diet?

10   Do you snack between meals?

11   When do you have your last meal of the day?

Is there anything else related to your lifestyle that could be of use to the trainer when designing an exercise programme?

Figure 3.7 Example lifestyle questionnaire (for a blank template visit: www.bloomsbury.com/9781408187234).

Table 3.3 Perceived barriers and potential solutions

Perceived barrier	Potential solutions
Time – such as work/family commitments	Design work-based activities. Get client to do family-based activities.
Injury	Depending on the injury other parts of the body can still be trained and in some situations non-impact fitness programme such as swimming could be prescribed.
Cost – facility or equipment	Design home or outdoor activities. Any clothing can be adapted. Break down the client perception that they need to follow trends.
Access – getting to facility	Sometimes clients are not even aware of certain facilities. Consider buddy-training or working out bus routes. Otherwise design home or outdoor activities.
Age	All fitness levels are relevant. Show client research and examples of how exercise can give benefits regardless of age, and stress the importance of reducing the risk of mortality.
Poor self-image	Discourage the client focusing on 'ideal body types'. Introduce to like-minded peer groups.
Lack of enjoyment	This could derive from a previous negative experience. Use testimonials to emphasise the fun factor of exercise.

If the client was not able to meet the process goal, this could potentially impact on the client achieving the outcome goal.

BARRIERS TO ACHIEVING GOALS

Individuals often cite many reasons for not adhering to an exercise programme. These cited 'reasons' are more commonly known as 'barriers to exercise'. Any barriers that cannot be overcome for genuine reasons such as illness and accidents are known as 'real barriers' whereas those that can be overcome by using appropriate strategies are known as 'perceived barriers'. Table 3.3 shows examples of perceived barriers and potential solutions. By identifying potential barriers in introductory client sessions (especially at the pre-contemplation and contemplation stages), appropriate strategies can be employed to help overcome the barriers and even eliminate them. Removing barriers means there is a greater chance of clients adopting and maintaining regular physical activity.

Gathering information relating to goals and barriers can be relatively straightforward if the trainer follows a simple process by standardising any questionnaires and information that they gather. Figure 3.7 is an example of a questionnaire (for a blank template please visit: www.bloomsbury.

com/9781408187234) that can be used to gather the information and subsequently record appropriate goals. The template allows the trainer to record the stage of change of the client (which should have been identified by using the Stage of Change questionnaire) as well as any strategies that might be related to that stage (see figure 3.1). The trainer should also estimate the level of self-efficacy of the client (see figure 3.6) so that they can make informed decisions about setting specific goals.

GOAL SETTING QUESTIONNAIRE

Client name

Date

Stage of change: Preparation

Self-efficacy level: 58

Client – please write down any goals that you would like to achieve in the....

Short-term:
Take part in aerobics sessions.

Medium-term:
Lose body fat

Long-term:
Maintain the loss

Agreed goals

Process:
Enrol in aerobics class twice weekly for first month. Increase to 3 times after that. Design resistance programme 2–3 sessions/week.

Outcome:
Target loss of 0.5kg/week with mid-term loss of 15kg (ideal weight). Maintain loss at 1-year review.

Client: please write down any barriers to taking part in exercise that you can think of:

Worried about what people think I look like. Difficulty getting to gym.

Solutions

Introduce to buddy (other client in similar position). Possibility of sharing transport.

Trainer – identify how you will make the programme SMART
- Specific: Weight loss
- Measurable: Short and long-term target in kg.
- Adjustable: Increase or decrease based on weekly measurement.
- Realistic: In line with current guidelines.
- Time based: Weekly for short-term leading to 30-week medium-term goal with maintenance for longer term.

Trainer – note any potential strategies related to stages of change:
- Include client in goal setting targets and accompany to gym to book aerobics sessions. Introduce to 'buddy'.

Figure 3.8 Example of a Goal Setting Questionnaire

Table 3.4	**Example of SMARTER goals**	
S	Specific	If an individual wants a weight-loss programme, be specific about the amount of weight that is set as the target. For instance, 0.5kg per week.
M	Measurable	In the example above, 0.5kg is a measurable amount as opposed to 'lose a little weight' each week.
A	Adjustable	If an individual finds the target too easy or too hard, then the trainer must adapt the programme to suit; in other words the programme must be adjustable.
R	Realistic	Set targets that are achievable. 0.5kg weight loss per week is an achievable target for most people whereas a target of 3kg per week might not be achievable by all people.
T	Time-based	0.5kg weight loss per week can be a short-term target that could lead to an overall loss of about 26kg a year, which is a long-term goal.

As you can see on the goal setting question-naire trainers should record how their goals relate to the SMART principle.

THE SMART PRINCIPLE

When agreeing goals with the client, whether short, medium or long-term, the acronym SMART – Specific, Measurable, Adjustable, Realistic and Time-based – is useful to keep in mind and each concept is associated with effective goal setting (see table 3.4). By using this principle, clients can be involved in the process and clearly visualise the agreed outcome in terms of specific goals and any strategies to be used.

IDENTIFY HEALTH AND FITNESS COMPONENTS

Once the trainer has set goals, they should follow this up with the appropriate health and fitness components, which could include specific fitness activities for sports-related goals, cardio for losing weight, and nutrition advice. Trainers should only select those components they feel qualified and experienced to deal with. As many health-related component tests require specialised equipment, there is often associated costs that go with them. Table 3.5 shows a comprehensive list of potential health components that trainers may choose to test (and monitor) with a list of associated testing equipment and their cost. The information related to health and fitness testing is broad ranging and not without debate and therefore beyond the scope of this book. For a more in-depth view please refer to *Practical Fitness Testing* by Coulson and Archer.

The ACSM lists the following as components of fitness: cardiovascular endurance, muscular strength, muscular endurance, flexibility, body composition and motor skills.

CARDIOVASCULAR ENDURANCE

Cardiovascular endurance, sometimes known as aerobic capacity, is the ability of the heart and lungs to deliver oxygen to the working muscles and for the muscles to use this oxygen to generate

Table 3.5 Health-related components, associated tests, equipment and costs

Health area	Test	Equipment needed	Approx cost
Heart rate	Palpation	None	None
	Telemetry	Heart rate monitor	£30–100
Body fat %	BMI	Stadiometer Scales	£60–1000; £20–500
	Skinfold	Callipers	£15–150
	Electrical impedance	Impedance tester	£150
Blood pressure	Pressure cuff	Sphygmomanometer	£20–200
Lung function	Forced Vital Capacity	Spirometer	£60–1,500
	Forced Expiratory Volume	Spirometer	
	Peak Expiratory Flow	Peak flow meter	£10–15
	Exercise Induced Bronchoconstriction	Spirometer	

work. It is commonly measured as 'volume of oxygen' (VO_2), with VO_2max being the maximum amount of oxygen that can be delivered to, and used by, the working muscles. The units used to measure VO_2 are millilitres of oxygen per kilogram of bodyweight per minute (mlO_2/kg/min or more scientifically as $mlO_2.kg^{-1}.min^{-1}$). In general terms, the best types of exercise for improving cardiovascular endurance are those that involve the use of large muscle groups: walking, hiking, running, stepping, swimming, cycling, dancing, skiing, skipping and so on.

MUSCULAR STRENGTH

This is the maximum amount of force that a muscle or muscle group can generate. Both static and dynamic muscular strength can be measured. In static strength testing, machines called dynamometers measure how much force an individual can exert against it without any movement. In dynamic strength testing, an individual moves an external load (usually free weights or resistance machines). This is known as repetition maximum testing or RM testing. 1RM is classed as the maximum amount of weight that can be lifted once with good form. It is possible to predict 1RM from multiple RM testing, for example, 6RM is the maximum amount of weight that can be lifted six times, which can then be used to predict 1RM. There are many methods of predicting 1RM (note that they are approximations) such as that proposed by Matt Brzycki (see box opposite).

$$1RM = \frac{W}{(1.0278 - (0.0278 \times r))}$$

W = the amount of weight lifted   r = the number of repetitions performed

Example: If a client had a 5RM of 80kg then:

$$1RM = \frac{80}{(1.0278 - (0.0278 \times 5))} = \frac{80}{(1.0278 - 0.139)} = \frac{80}{0.88} = 91KG$$

Muscular strength can be developed through resistance training, including using machine and free weights, body weight and resistance bands.

MUSCULAR ENDURANCE

Muscular endurance is ability of a muscle or muscle group to perform repeated contractions against resistance over a period of time. Muscular endurance is typical of low-level muscular contractions that need to be maintained for a period of time, such as that in stabilisation, and is associated with resistance training using relatively low intensity and high repetitions. Hypertrophy – the increase in cross-sectional diameter of skeletal muscle – is not usually associated with this type of training. Testing normally involves recording the maximum number of repetitions, such as push-ups or sit-ups.

FLEXIBILITY

This is the ability to move a joint through its complete range of motion. An individual may be flexible in one joint and not in another. Therefore, all joints must be assessed individually using 'goniometry', where the angle of each joint is measured and compared against tables for normal ranges of motion. A common flexibility test used in the health and fitness industry is the 'sit and reach' test, where an individual sits with straight legs and reaches forward. The distance reached with the fingertips is then recorded. This measures only hamstring and upper back flexibility and is often a topic of debate as to its validity, so other tests should also be carried out. There are several types of stretching exercise that improve flexibility including static, dynamic, PNF and ballistic.

BODY COMPOSITION

This refers to the ratio of fat to lean tissue in an individual: in other words, how lean, over-weight or obese a person is. Even though body composition is listed as a component of fitness, it is probably more accurate to associate it with an indication of health as excess body fat is associated with disease such as hypertension, diabetes, stroke, coronary heart disease and hyperlipidaemia. Although the causes of obesity can include hypothalamic, endocrine and genetic disorders, diet and physical inactivity are the prime factors. It is generally accepted and recommended by the ACSM that an increase in calorie expenditure and a decrease in calorie intake is the most effective long-term method for treating obesity: between 150 and 400 Kcal of daily energy expenditure is recommended for weight-loss programmes (for methods of how to measure overweight and obesity please refer to *Practical Fitness Testing* by Coulson and Archer).

MOTOR SKILLS

There are many sub-components of motor skills, including speed, power, agility, coordination and balance. All of these areas have been shown to improve with appropriate training.

- Speed is the ability to move quickly from one point to another and can be improved by specifically targeting variables such as muscle coordination, efficiency of body movement, core strength and flexibility.
- Power is a combination of strength and speed and can be developed through plyometric and resistance training.
- Agility is the ability to change direction at speed and is generally thought to improve as a result of speed and power training combined with agile specific movements.

Table 3.6 Components of health and fitness related to activities

Goal-related activity	Cardio	Muscular Strength	Muscular Endurance	Flex	Balance	Speed	Agility	Power
Aerobics								
Aqua								
Studio dance								
Cycling	✓		✓			✓		✓
Resistance training		✓	✓					✓
Running	✓	✓	✓	✓	✓	✓	✓	✓
Swimming								
Tai Chi								
Walking								
Yoga								

Heart rate	Body fat %	Blood pressure	Lung function
✓		✓	

- Balance is the ability to maintain equilibrium at all times. Proprioceptors in the body give information to the brain on the position of limbs, as well as balance information from the inner ear and the eyes. Most forms of balance training (from static to dynamic) will result in an improvement in balance.
- Coordination is the ability to move the limbs precisely in a particular direction.

Trainers should identify which components of fitness the client needs to work on, and the activities that we help them achieve their goals. For example, table 3.6 gives a list of common activities and the related components of fitness. Once the chosen activities are listed trainers should then identify which components of fitness are relevant to each activity by placing a tick in the appropriate column. The trainer should then decide which health-related components should be included by ticking the appropriate boxes in the bottom row.

Using a template such as that in table 3.6 allows the trainer to synthesise a great deal of information into a simple and easy to read format which can be kept as a reference.

Having completed the health and fitness component profile, trainers would then need to decide which components of fitness were of primary importance for the client and which were secondary. It's necessary to do this as it would be unrealistic for the trainer to target all components of fitness at the same time. Many experienced trainers would be able to do this without much help but those trainers new to this type of analysis could use a simple components of fitness importance check-sheet such as the example in table 3.7.

Table 3.7	Components of fitness importance check-sheet		
	Importance of component		
	Hi	**Med**	**Lo**
Cardio endurance	✓		
Muscular strength			✓
Muscular endurance		✓	
Flexibility		✓	
Balance	✓		
Speed		✓	
Agility	✓		
Power		✓	

Comments:
- Flexibility – concentrate on hamstring and hip flexors.
- Speed – focus on acceleration component.
- Power – jump ability is important.

The check-sheets above have been done for a client, an amateur football player, who wants to improve his fitness levels. Keep in mind that this type of analysis is subjective and different trainers might not agree with what is considered to be high, medium or low in terms of the importance of fitness components for a particular activity. By completing the checklist the trainer would then be able to make an informed decision as to which fitness tests were then suitable.

TEST COMPONENTS

One of the many objectives related to health and fitness testing is to establish a comprehensive physiological profile of an individual at the start of the process. If levels of certain health and fitness components are established as a result of testing, a more detailed and accurate exercise programme can be designed with a view to re-testing after a period of training to measure how successful the programme has been. If done correctly, health and fitness testing can also have many other benefits to both trainer and client as can be seen in table 3.8.

The range and choice of fitness tests available to the trainer is huge and beyond the scope of this book and, again, all tests can be found in *Practical Fitness Testing* (Coulson and Archer). However, figure 3.9 gives an example of typical physiological fitness tests that are carried out in a personal training environment. The physiological fitness test includes a column that relates to the component of health and fitness, a column which shows the units that each test is measured in, and a column that gives the target ranges relating to men or women based on normative data from specific age ranges. Any tests that are first carried out for a client are known as 'baseline tests' as they provide details of the client's components of health and fitness at that particular time. All subsequent testing is then usually referred to as 'follow-up' testing.

Table 3.8	Benefits of health and fitness testing
Benefit of testing	**Description of benefit**
Identify strengths and weaknesses	Testing can help to establish an overall picture of the client's physical condition. It also provides baseline data for individual training programmes and can help to assess the health status of clients which can act as a potential monitor for overtraining.
Monitor progress	By repeating tests at specific intervals the effectiveness of the training programme can be monitored. Results also provide a useful motivational tool to encourage clients.
Grouping	If the trainer is working with a group of clients, then testing can provide information which allows grouping of individuals according to ability.
Education	Testing can help to provide a better understanding of the demands of the particular sport or event for both the trainer and the client.
Recovery guide	Testing is a very useful way to assess recovery from injury and readiness for training.
Motivation	Baseline results can be used to set standards and motivate clients towards the next testing session.
Goal setting	Both short- and long-term objectives can be established based on test results.

Before any tests are carried out, trainers must get the consent of the client in writing, having fully explained to them the nature of the chosen tests. This can be done using a Health & Fitness Assessment Consent Form (for a blank template please visit: www.bloomsbury.com/9781408187234). Trainers should make sure the client fully understands the form before they sign it and then they should keep the form (as per Data Protection Act procedures) for as long as they are working with the client and for a period of time afterwards.

Body data, body composition, blood pressure, lung function and flexibility are known as 'health or static tests' as they do not require any physical exertion by the subject being tested. The other tests are known as 'fitness or dynamic tests'. It is useful when carrying out multiple tests to record the results using some form of standardised recording mechanism (see figure 3.9). This record should then be kept for future reference. As the record will include personal information, treat it as confidential and keep it in lockable storage with restricted access. The date of the testing procedure undertaken should always be recorded to compare against subsequent tests (although this is goal dependent a period of 12 weeks is common between testing procedures). This can be used as a basis on which to justify any programme adjustment or alteration decisions. Figure 3.11 shows an example of a typical assessment sheet that can easily be adapted by trainers.

As can be seen on the assessment sheet there is a column marked 'category'. Trainers can use this column to compare tests results with normative data tables that are published for many common tests (these are readily available on the internet and can easily be found by searching for normative values for the relevant test). Depending on the test result, normative data tables often give a categorisation for the score related to performance, such as: below average, average and above average. The comments column could be used to note certain details such as time of day; environment, problems and how the client was feeling at the time of the test.

CYCLICAL TESTING PROCESS

The process of baseline testing and follow-up testing can be thought of in cyclical terms as shown in figure 3.10. Irrespective of the method of testing to be carried out, the cyclical process provides the trainer with a standardised and easy to follow format as follows:

1. **Select characteristics to be measured**
   This simply means deciding which particular components of health and fitness are to be tested.

2. **Select appropriate measuring tool**
   Once a range of components have been determined (for example, strength, aerobic capacity, flexibility, etc), the correct protocol can be established depending on the availability of resources to the trainer.

3. **Collect data**
   Test results can then be collected having followed the correct test protocol. It should be remembered that all data is confidential.

4. **Analyse collected data**
   The data can then be analysed and interpreted by first putting it into the correct format and then comparing against either previous test data or population data (for example, how does the score compare against the population in terms of being in a category of poor to excellent). Analysis of test results becomes easier as

Component	Test	Units	Target range	Comments
Body data	Height	cm	See BMI	
	Weight	kg	See BMI	
	Heart rate	bpm		Men18–35yrs average = 66–69 Women 18–35yrs average = 68–71
Body composition	BMI	Index score	<25	Overweight 25-29.9 Obese ≥ 30
	Skinfold	Fat %	M: <25% F: <30%	Skinfolds in millimetres converted to fat %
	Electrical impedance	Fat %	M: <25% F: <30%	Adhere to pre-test conditions
Blood pressure	Manual blood pressure	mmHg	120/80 <140/90	Normal = 120/80 Hypertension = 140/90
Lung function	FVC	L		Refer to height/age related tables
	FEV1	L		Refer to height/age related tables
	EIB	% drop	<10% drop	Mild = 10–24% drop
Flexibility	Sit & reach test	cm	M: ≥22cm F: ≥22cm	Male adults average = 22–25 Female adults average 22–26
	Modified sit & reach	cm	M: ≥14.4cm F: ≥14.8cm	Male adults average = 14.4 Female adults average = 14.8
Cardio endurance	Multi-stage fitness test	level	M: level ≥7 F: level ≥6	Male adults average = 7–9 Female adults average = 6–8
	Cooper 12-minute run	m		Age-related scores
	Rockport walk test	bpm s		Aim to set a baseline and improve
Balance	Stork test	s	≥25s	Adults average = 25–39

Power	Vertical jump	cm	M: ≥41cm	Male adults average = 41–50
			F: ≥31cm	Female adults average = 31–40
	30m sprint	s	M: ≤4.4s	Male adults average = 4.3–4.4
			F: ≤4.7s	Female adults average = 4.7–4.8
Agility	Illinois agility test	s	M: ≤18.1s	Male adults average = 16.2–18.1
			F: ≤21.7s	Female adults average = 18–21.7
Muscular strength/ endurance	Multiple rep max	kg		Aim to set a baseline and improve
Core stability	TA contraction	mmHg	-2 to -6	Bio-pressure feedback unit to measure drop in pressure on contraction of TA

Figure 3.9 Typical Physiological Assessments

the trainer gains more experience with administering the particular tests.

5. **Adjustment to programme**
This part of the cycle is not relevant to baseline testing but is useful for all subsequent follow-up tests. Having interpreted the results, adjustments to the training programme can be made based on the judgement of the success of the programme to-date.

6. **Agree follow-up test date**
Regular testing should be carried out in order to establish the success of the programme as measured by the components being tested. The duration between tests should be long enough to allow adaptation as a result of training but should be short enough to provide information to adapt the programme and also set achievable goals. It is often the case that changes must be made in relation to the lifestyle commitments of the client but changes should also be

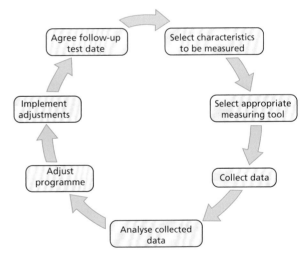

Figure 3.10 Cyclical testing process

made if the trainer feels that the client is not 'on-track' to achieve the set goals. Therefore the importance of regular testing can never be underestimated as it provides the trainer (and client) with valuable and varied information.

HEALTH AND FITNESS ASSESSMENT SHEET

Test	Score	Category	Test	Score	Category	Comments
Blood Pressure	Syst Dias		Balance	s		
EIB	% drop		Vertical jump	cm		
Body fat	%		Walk test	Time VO_2		
Sit and reach	cm		Step test	bpm VO_2		
Heart rate	bpm		MSFT	Level VO_2		
Lung function	FVC FEV1 PF		Cooper 12-min walk	m VO_2		
BMI	Height Weight		Agility	s		
x RM	Chest Leg		30m sprint	s		
Core stability	± mmhg					

Client name

Tester name

Date

Figure 3.11 Health and fitness assessment sheet (for a template visit: www.bloomsbury.com/9781408187234).

PROGRAMME DESIGN

4

THE NOS LEVEL 3 PERSONAL TRAINER CRITERIA COVERED IN THIS CHAPTER ARE:

- How to research and identify exercises and activities to help clients to achieve their goals
- How to identify accepted good practice in designing personal training programmes
- How to apply the principles of training to programme design
- How to design a progressive programme to allow your clients to achieve short-, medium- and longterm goals
- How to monitor and adapt a client's adherence strategy
- How to choose resources and environments that will help your clients to participate in the programme according to their needs
- How to design programmes that can be run in environments not designed for physical exercise, for example, a client's home or outdoor area
- How to decide on the order of exercises and activities in the programme
- Current guidelines on programme design and safe exercise
- How to make sure the components of fitness are built into the programme
- How to structure and record the sessions which make up the programme
- Why it is important to agree the programme with your clients
- When it is appropriate to share the programme with other professionals
- Why it is important for the client to take responsibility for their own fitness/behaviour change
- What types of issues may need to be referred to another professional, when to refer them and who this professional may be in different situations
- The importance of explaining any delay in dealing with clients and how to do so effectively

PERSONAL TRAINING

PROGRAMME DESIGN

In terms of occupational competence, one of the main differences between a level 2 trainer and a PT is that the latter is expected to design individual programmes to meet clients' needs. This means that each client programme should be carefully planned, but as goals and needs often change, it is important that the trainer reflects after each session so that any programmes can be adapted if needed.

The knowledge required to design appropriate individual programmes should be broad and in-depth so trainers should constantly keep up to date with research relating to diet and exercise interventions and keep abreast of current thinking in the area of exercise prescription. There are many credible sources of information that the trainer can access in relation to guidelines (mentioned throughout this book) that have been established as a result of evidence of best practice

and, as such, have a history of success. Regardless of the programme to be designed, certain fundamental principles should always be applied when designing an individual programme of exercise.

PRINCIPLES OF FITNESS

When designing any exercise programme it is important to remember that certain fundamental factors can have an effect on the outcome of the programme. These factors are called 'principles of fitness'. These principles must be taken into account with all clients in relation to the design of a training or exercise programme.

Specificity

The body can adapt to the demands of various types of exercise, and the type of adaptation that takes place is dependent on the muscle fibres involved and the frequency, intensity and duration of the exercises. For example, type 1 fibres will

Table 4.1	ACSM FITT guidelines for exercise		
	Cardio	**Resistance**	**Flexibility**
Frequency	3–5 days per week.	2–3 non-consecutive sessions per week.	Minimum 2–3 sessions per week, ideally 5–7 sessions per week.
Intensity	55–90% of maximum heart rate (RPE 12–16).	1 set of 3–20 repetitions to volitional fatigue while maintaining good form (RPE 16–20).	To the end range of motion at a point of tightness, without pain.
Time	20–60 minutes continuous or intermittent aerobic exercise.	Enough to carry out 8–10 separate exercises for total body.	15–30 seconds (2–4 times for each stretch)
Type	Large muscle mass, rhythmic, aerobic	Body weight, machines, free-weights, bands	Static, preceded by a warm-up.

50

adapt to endurance training, while type 2 fibres will adapt to more intense strength training. The body will also adapt to the type (or specificity) of the training. For example, an individual who trains predominantly on a treadmill will become better at using the treadmill even though there will be a certain transfer of fitness to other types of cardio exercise. This is sometimes referred to as the SAID principle – Specific Adaptation to Imposed Demands. Trainers should try and match the type of training to the client's goals, taking into account the likes and dislikes of the client. The guidelines relating to frequency, intensity, duration and type most often used in the industry are those of the American College of Sports Medicine (2009) as shown in table 4.1.

Adaptation

This principle states that the adaptations derived from an exercise are specific to the exercise and to the muscles involved. For example, runners show little improvement in the muscular endurance of their arm muscles, while cyclists show most of their muscular endurance improvement in their leg muscles. In order for adaptation in the body to occur, however, the body must be subjected to the exercise on a regular basis.

Overload

In order for an individual to adapt to a new demand or routine, overload must be achieved. Overload can be described as 'taking the body or system to a point just beyond what it is usually accustomed to' (ACSM, 2009). If any system within the body (a muscle or an organ) is made to work harder than it normally does on a regular basis, it will undergo certain physical changes to adapt. It is important to remember that the body

should be taken to a workload just beyond normal levels; if it is taken too far, injury may occur. There are many ways in which overload can be achieved within a programme in order to progress to achieve adaptation. Length, speed, resistance and gravity are among many variables in which to progress a programme of exercise.

Progression

If the workload of a training programme does not progress, the individual will not continue to adapt. Instead, once the body has adapted to the current workload, it will not attempt to adapt any further. In order to progress, the workload must be periodically changed once the body has become accustomed to the previous workload. The rate of progression is specific to each individual and can also be affected by various factors:

- Fitness level: less fit individuals will progress at a faster rate than fitter individuals.
- Experience: an individual with past experience of certain exercises will progress at a faster rate than those with no experience.
- Injury: an injury to a specific site can reverse any gains previously made at that site. It is important to remember that the rest of the body may be trained to prevent total body reversibility.
- Environment: the nature of the environment can affect progression in several ways. For example, altitude training can have an effect on oxygen transport, while heat and cold can affect the rate of progression.

Progression should be considered during the design stage of the programme. This way, progression can be focused on short-, medium- and long-term goals. It is the role of the trainer to monitor the client during each session in order to determine if they are ready to progress with each component of fitness as the plan dictates. A regular schedule of testing will also help trainers to make this judgement. If the client is not ready to progress as scheduled, then the plan should be adapted.

Regression (reversibility)

Just as the body can become stronger if the workload is increased, the body can become weaker over a period of time if the workload is reduced. It is possible for specific fitness components to diminish within two weeks of cessation of exercise. This principle is known as regression.

Individuality

As all clients progress at different rates due to their genetic make-up, it is important that frequency, intensity and duration of exercise are manipulated to suit the client. In any health-related fitness programme, clients should be encouraged to start slowly and begin at levels that can easily be maintained. Progression should then be encouraged when the client feels that he or she can cope with the current workload and is able to progress.

Recovery time

One thing that is often missing from a progressive training programme is recovery time. It is obvious that rest is an important component of any exercise programme, as are active recovery periods (for example, very low intensity aerobic exercise). Trainers should constantly monitor clients for signs of exhaustion and over-training (see page 62) such as drop in performance, increase in resting heart rate and regular illness. Recovery of the muscular, cardiovascular and neural systems depend on many factors such as the intensity of the training session, individual fitness levels, age, psychological factors and dietary interventions. As a very general guideline, clients should be given a 24- to 48-hour recovery period following a bout of exercise. However, this can be split according to the body area/muscle group, so that training can take place each day. With resistance training, for example, daily sessions could take place but different muscle groups could be targeted on different days to allow recovery.

Lifestyle

What a client does on a daily basis has a major effect on their fitness level. For example in 2002, a report from the World Health Organization (WHO) stated that physical inactivity (less than 2.5 hours per week of moderate intensity activity or 1 hour per week of vigorous activity) is one of the ten leading causes of death in developed countries, resulting in more than 1.9 million deaths worldwide per year. For this reason it is imperative that trainers encourage an active lifestyle and should therefore consider other activities, over and above those they are designing, that clients would like to participate in. These activities can be incorporated into the training programme, for example: swim training sessions contributing to the overall cardio fitness component are considered as part of the weekly plan.

If a client is under the guidance of any other professional such as a coach or physiotherapist, then the trainer should make every attempt to liaise and communicate with the other professional to figure out how the programme integrates with any other training sessions and goals. If trainers consider alternative activities, then they must take into account the resources required and also the environment in which the activities could take place.

- Resources: the resources available to the trainer relate to small equipment that can be purchased, such as kettle bells, stability balls, medicine balls, boxing gloves/pads, resistance bands and weighted vests, etc. or equipment that would only be available in facilities, such as cardio machines, resistance equipment, punch bags, swimming pool, etc. Some trainers prefer to collaborate with facilities in order to access equipment however; investing in a variety of small equipment that is transportable can increase the range of clients that can be targeted.
- Environment: there are a range of environments in which the client can train, such as fitness facilities, the trainer's home or studio, the client's home and outdoors. The environment/s that the client prefers should be discussed during the initial consultation so that relevant resources can then be selected to suit the particular environment. Regardless of the environment chosen, trainers should always carry out a risk assessment (see page 213) to make sure that the environment is suitable for training purposes.

EXERCISE ORDER

A typical exercise session as recommended by the American College of Sports Medicine would include:

1. Warm-up
2. Conditioning phase (including cardio, resistance and flexibility training)
3. Cool-down.

Within the conditioning phase the cardio session (if not too intense) could be done prior to the resistance session or the resistance session could be done first (again if not too intense). The trainer

Table 4.2	The ABCs exercise order

A Agonist – antagonist
Training an agonist (the muscle doing the work) followed by its antagonist (the muscle opposing the agonist) seems to have beneficial effects and also helps to achieve muscular balance, which can help to reduce the risk of injury.

B Big to small
Train larger muscle groups before smaller muscles groups. If doing an exercise that involves both and the smaller muscle group is fatigued, this will impact on the larger muscle group.

C Compound to isolation
Exercises that involve multi-joint coordination (typically free-weights) should be done prior to isolated joint exercises (typically resistance machines).

S Stabilisation last
Similar to the big-to-small principle, train stabilisers last as it is not effective to fatigue stabilisers first as they will be required for all other exercises.

should consider the alternative of doing resistance and cardio on separate days if planned sessions are intense. In terms of the order of resistance exercises there are many factors that could impact on the decision. It is recommended that the trainer follow a simple principle such as the ABCs exercise order as shown in table 4.2.

There has been a vast amount of research into building stretches into the programme. Consensus of opinion appears to support prescribing dynamic type stretches prior to the main cardio or resistance session and static type stretches afterwards. For more information on advanced training techniques please read *The Advanced Fitness Trainers Handbook* by Coulson and Archer. Taking into account principles of fitness and exercise order, it is the role of the trainer to design an individual exercise programme by matching components of health and fitness to specific time-based goals. This process is more commonly known as 'periodisation'.

PERIODISATION

The term 'periodisation' is used in both sport and health and fitness. It relates to programme design and the process of manipulation of a programme of exercise at regular intervals, known as cycles. Although periodisation is used predominantly by athletes in order to organise their training programmes so that they 'peak' at competition times, it is also used in the health and fitness industry as the regular manipulation of an exercise programme is thought to elicit optimal gains in one or more components of health and fitness. In order to achieve this, it is common to monitor on-going performance so that the programme can be adjusted accordingly depending on the nature of the results. The programme can be organised into intervals known as cycles whereby each cycle has a different time duration:

- **Microcycle:** this is the shortest interval within an exercise programme and normally refers to a seven-day period (that is, short-term planning). Any goals within such a short period of time need to be achievable in relation to the individual.
- **Mesocycle:** this is a repeating series of microcycles over a period of several weeks (that is, medium-term planning). The goals in a mesocycle should be achievable yet flexible, as they can be manipulated following analysis of the microcycles within it.
- **Macrocycle:** this is a series of mesocycles, normally over a period of a few months to several years (that is, long-term planning). Information gathered from microcycles and mesocycles can be used to confirm or readjust the long-term goals of the macrocycle. Each microcycle period should contribute to the goals of the mesocycles, which in turn will contribute to the goals of the overall macrocycle.

Planning a programme of exercise using periodised cycles can be useful as it can focus on individual short-, medium- and long-term goals. This has been shown to have a positive effect on adherence to exercise, not only for beginners but for regular exercisers as well. There are many ways of designing a periodised exercise programme but one of the more common methods is that of the step-loading model.

Mesocycle models

Simple progressive overload training programmes are often thought to be boring and repetitive for

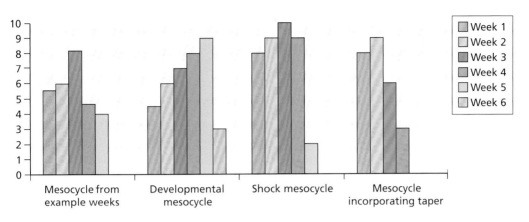

Figure 4.1 Illustration of various mesocycle used to develop a macrocycle

the individual, as well as leading to staleness and increasing the risk of repetitive loading injuries, therefore, there are many alternative ways in which to design and implement training programmes known as 'mesocycle models'. As can be seen in figure 4.1 a step-loading model normally includes two or three microcycles of increases in training intensity followed by cycles of decreased training intensity within the overall mesocycle.

A developmental mesocycle on the other hand is one in which there is a progressive intensity increase in the microcycle training sessions followed by a recovery microcyle at the end of the mesocycle. A shock mesocycle is one in which there are several high-intensity microcyles followed by a very low-intensity recovery microcycle and a tapering mesocycle is one in which the training intensity of the microcycles steadily decreases.

General Fitness Pyramid model

It is often difficult to decide which components of fitness should be developed first before progressing with a programme. As the goals and abilities of individuals is vastly different it is down to the skill and knowledge of the trainer; however, there is a general model that can be adopted which fits the majority of potential clients. This is known as the General Fitness Pyramid Model as in figure 4.2, which shows a progressive phase construction.

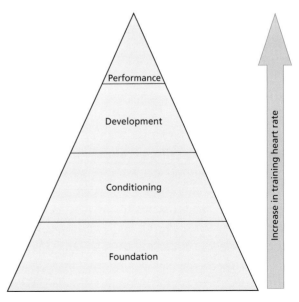

Figure 4.2 General Fitness Pyramid Model

- **Foundation:** As with any progressive model you need to provide a base foundation of fitness prior to progressing in any way. Typical fitness components that are targeted include flexibility, joint mobility (range of movement), joint stabilisation (posture awareness and static balance), and aerobic base fitness.
- **Development:** Once the trainer is satisfied that the client has achieved a reasonable level of the foundation components they should then concentrate on developing components such as movement coordination, dynamic balance and stability and aerobic conditioning.
- **Conditioning:** Depending on the goals of the client the following components could then be developed: Muscular strength/endurance, hypertrophy, agility, anaerobic and aerobic capacity.
- **Performance:** For those clients who have specific performance goals the following components should then be developed: Power, speed, skill (if appropriate), aerobic and anaerobic capacity.

Once clients achieve a certain level of fitness after progressing through the foundation and development phases, trainers should carefully consider how to structure training sessions for the conditioning and performance phases in relation to cardiovascular and muscular ability. If the client is training for a particular sport, then the training should complement that sport. For example, distance rowing and swimming would require a focus on cardiovascular and muscular endurance whereas boxing and martial arts would require a combination of muscular power and muscular endurance as well as aerobic and anaerobic capacity.

Regardless of the periodisation model used, it is important for the trainer to have a visual plan of individual training sessions and how these fit into an overall long-term period of training. There are many ways in which to do this but one simple method is that of reverse planning using a macro-cycle planning sheet. The example shown in figure 4.4 has been completed for a fictitious sub-elite sprint swimmer using the details in figure 4.3.

CLIENT DETAILS:

Gender: Male

Age: 23

Weight: 79kg

Height: 186cm

Client has reasonable experience of using the gym although he has never been on an athlete programme and has always trained on his own. He is very enthusiastic about dry-land training in order to help his swimming performance. He has a full timetable as far as swim training is concerned and only has one full rest day per week.

CLIENT OBJECTIVES:

He feels he needs more strength, especially in his abdominal region and upper body. He wants a fuller chest and wants to improve strength in his arms and chest as he feels they are his weak point. He has never trained his legs before and isn't sure if adding muscle to them would affect his swimming. He feels fit when sprint swimming but feels that dry land cardio work would help his sprint endurance.

Figure 4.3

MACROCYCLE

Main goals: Increase aerobic and anaerobic endurance. Develop upper body strength and core stabilisation. Maintain flexibility and body composition.

Tests: VO_2max (aerobic endurance). Onset Blood Lactate (anaerobic endurance). 5RM (strength). TA contraction (core stability). Sit and reach (flexibility). Skinfolds (body composition).

	Jan				Feb				March				April		
	Week				Week				Week				Week		
1	2	3	4	1	2	3	4	1	2	3	4	1	2	3	4

MESOCYCLES

Foundation	Development	Conditioning	Performance
• Baseline testing before week 1. • Introduce core stabilisation and flexibility exercises. • Introduce cardio training (aerobic). • Assess resistance training ability and start with light weights to develop ligament strength.	• Increase volume of core stability exercises. • Increase cardio volume. • Build up volume and intensity of weights for hypertrophy. • Develop flexibility as required.	• Re-test end of week 4. • Increase challenge of core stability exercises. • Introduce anaerobic to support aerobic programme. • Increase intensity of weights and decrease volume. • Maintain flexibility.	• Progress to using stability ball as the bench and introduce plyometric upper body exercises. • Interval training at approximate swim distance times. • Maintain flexibility.

MICROCYCLES

Wk 1	Wk 2	Wk 3	Wk 4	Wk 1	Wk 2	Wk 3	Wk 4	Wk 1	Wk 2	Wk 3	Wk 4	Wk 1	Wk 2	Wk 3	Wk 4
CS1	CS1	CS1	CS1	CS1/2	CS1/2	CS1/2	CS1/2	CS2/3	CS2/3	CS2/3	CS2/3	CS1/4	CS1/4	CS1/4	CS1/4
UB1	UB1	UB1	UB1	UB1/2	UB1/2	UB1/2	UB1/2	UB1/2	UB1/2	UB1/2	UB1/2	WB	WB	WB	WB
LB1	LB1	LB1	LB1	LB1/2	LB1/2	LB1/2	LB1/2	LB1/2	LB1/2	LB1/2	LB1/2				

CS = Cardio session UB = Upper body LB = Lower body WB = Whole body
NB: Flexibility sessions dependent on testing

Specificity	Adaptation	Overload	Progression	Regression	Individuality	Recovery
= p	= p	= p	= p	= p	= p	= p

Figure 4.4 Example macrocycle plan for a sub-elite swimmer

PROGRAMME DESIGN

57

When using this method the trainer should first record the overall goals for the macrocycle period (in this case approximately four months). Once this has been done the trainer can then develop more specific objectives for each mesocycle (typically a period of a month). This particular method allows for the components of the General Fitness Pyramid Model to be incorporated as shown in the example in figure 4.4 (for a blank template please visit: www.bloomsbury.com/9781408187234) whereby goals for the foundation, development, conditioning and performance stages have been set in relation to the overall macrocycle goals. Information from the Goal Setting Questionnaire (see page 38) can

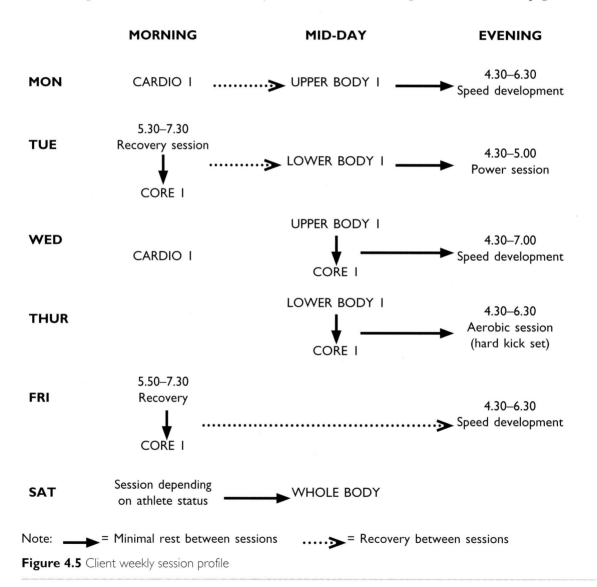

Figure 4.5 Client weekly session profile

be used to help develop both the mesocycle and macrocycle goals. Finally microcycles (typically one week) can be planned with information relating to individual component training sessions. As can be seen in the example, each microcycle of one week contains cardio and resistance training codes (i.e. CS, UB, LB and WB) which relate to individual training sessions that are planned separately. Before each individual session is planned it is advisable to map out a weekly session profile of the client in order to identify when each session will take place. This will need to be done in consultation with the client for the purpose of accuracy of information and agreement.

Figure 4.5 shows an example of a typical weekly profile for the swimmer with all individual sessions incorporated. In this particular case the swimming sessions are already in place therefore the other training sessions have to be incorporated to fit around those sessions. Each individual session can then be planned and recorded as shown. For example, figure 4.6 shows the individual sessions for resistance training and core stabilisation (for a blank template please visit: www.bloomsbury.com/9781408187234) whereas figure 4.7 shows the cardiovascular training sessions. Information relating to the weight lifted for each resistance exercise would be ascertained during initial induction sessions, as would cardiovascular intensity if trainers prefer the use of heart-rate monitors. Note that the bottom row of the macrocycle planning sheet includes principles of fitness that can be ticked if

MICROCYCLE RECORD SHEET

Client name

Mesocycle   Microcycle week

	Exercise	Intensity (RM)	Comment
Upper Body 1	Bent Over Row	3 SETS (14, 14, 12)	Keep neutral spine and tension in TA.
	Db Chest Press – Bench	3 SETS (14, 14, 12)	Limit decent so upper arm parallel with floor.
	Db Shoulder Press	3 SETS (14, 14, 12)	Db no lower than shoulder level.
	Tricep Over Head (Double)	3 SETS (12, 10, 10)	Keep forearm in swimming position.
	Db Bicep Curl (Single)	3 SETS (14, 14, 12)	Avoid twisting motion.
	Shoulder Internal/External Rotation	3 SETS (16, 16, 14)	Maintain neutral spine.
Upper Body 2	Cable Cross Flye Standing	3 SETS (14, 14, 12)	Alternate between split and square stance.
	Single Arm Cable Pull Through	3 SETS (14, 14, 12)	Mimic swim motion.
	Seated Row	3 SETS (14, 14, 12)	Use horizontal handles and keep elbows high.
	Shoulder Shrug	3 SETS (14, 14, 12)	No rotation.

Figure 4.6 Microcycle record sheet for resistance and core stabilisation training

Upper Body 3	Plyometric Push Ups	3 SETS (14, 14, 12)	Stop if form lost.
	Plometric Standing Med Ball Chest Throw	3 SETS (14, 14, 12)	Keep neutral spine throughout.
	Supine Med Ball Overhead Throw	3 SETS (14, 14, 12)	Keep bend in knees.
Legs 1	Alternating: Squat and Bounding	5 SETS (12, 10, 10, 12, 12) 5 SETS of 40 metres	Full ROM. Contract TA. Quick land-to-take-off phase.
	Alternating: Split Squat and Box Jump	5 SETS (12, 10, 10, 12, 12) 5 SETS (6)	Set on one leg then set on the other.
Legs 2	Alternating: Single Leg Db Squat and Hopping	5 SETS (12, 10, 10, 12, 12) 5 SETS of 30 metres	Use a low bench but maintain posture. Quick land-to-take-off phase.
	Alternating: Dead Lift and Lunge Drops	5 SETS (12, 10, 10, 12, 12) 5 SETS (6 each leg)	Contract TA and keep neutral spine. Keep posture at all times.
Whole Body	Power Cleans	3 SETS (12, 12, 10)	Stop if form lost.
	Split Cleans	3 SETS (12, 12, 10)	Stop if form lost.
	Wood Choppers	3 SETS (12, 12, 10)	Stop if form lost.
	Med Ball Scoops	3 SETS (12, 10, 8)	Face down on bench. Scoop ball in swim action.
Core 1	Supine Foot Slide	All stability exercises to be done to fatigue or loss of form.	There are many sources for core stabilisation exercises.
	Supine Knee Rolls		
	Superman		
Core 2	Foot Bridge Roll		
	Front Bridge Rolls		
Core 3	Shoulder Med Ball Drop		
	Kneeling Med Ball Throws		
Core 4	Single Arm Row (Ball as bench)		
	Cable Cross Flye – Swiss Ball		
	Swiss Ball Hip Crunch		
	Swiss Ball Hamstring Curls		

Figure 4.6 Microcycle record sheet for resistance and core stabilisation training (*cont.*)

MICROCYCLE RECORD SHEET

Client name

Mesocycle   Microcycle week

	Exercise	Intensity (RPR 1–10)	Comment
CARDIO 1	Warm-up: 3-5 mins cycle/rower	3–6	The length of the main session depends on the ability of the client. Monitor this closely.
	Main: 20–30 mins treadmill	6–8	
	Cool-down: 3-5 mins cycle	8–3	
CARDIO 2	Warm-up: 3-5 mins cycle/rower	3–6	Increase the duration of the main session by about 15-20%.
	Main: 25–35 mins treadmill	6–8	
	Cool-down: 3-5 mins cycle	8–3	
CARDIO 3	Warm-up: 3-5 mins cycle/rower	3–6	Introduce periods of higher intensity. This is designed to take the client just into the anaerobic zone. Do not go to max at this stage.
	Main: 5–10 mins	6–8	
	10–12 mins	8–9	
	12–20 mins	9–6–8	
	20–22 mins	8–9	
	22–35 mins	9–6–8	
	Cool-down:	8–3	
CARDIO 4	Warm-up: 5–10 mins	3–6	Number of high intensity intervals depends on ability of client. After each interval reduce intensity quickly then slowly build up in the next 4 minute period.
	Main: 5–10 mins	6–8	
	10–11 mins	8–10	
	11–15 mins	10–7	
	15–16 mins	7–10	
	16–20 mins	10–7	
	21–22 mins	7–10	
	Cool-down: 5–10 mins	10–3	

Figure 4.7 Microcycle record sheet for cardio training

61

they are taken into consideration when planning the programme. These principles will be discussed in more detail in chapter 8. Once an individual programme has been designed for a particular client, the client and the programme must then be accurately monitored on a regular basis for several reasons. As mentioned in the section on testing, regular monitoring is essential for determining the suitability of the programme for the client at that particular time. As well as this, monitoring is also essential in order to determine the physiological and psychological state of the client in relation to over-reaching and over-training.

OVER-TRAINING

Anecdotally, one of the main problems associated with clients taking part in regular exercise programmes is that of 'over-training'. The term 'over-training' is generally considered to relate to a physiological and psychological state brought about by an excessive amount of training over a long period of time. The term 'over-reaching' tends to be used for similar situations but related to occurrence in the short-term. In other words, over-reaching can lead to over-training if it is not dealt with effectively. Some researchers question the evidence for over-training and also whether over-reaching can actually lead to over-training (Halson and Jeukendrup, 2004), however, it is common for athletes to report experiencing over-training at some stage in their career. Although it is difficult to diagnose and not without contention, there are considered to be several common signs of over-training, such as those indicated in table 4.3 that the trainer should be aware of.

If over-training symptoms are evident, trainers should suggest that the training load of the client be reduced until they have recovered enough to start training again. With clients who are often reluctant to rest for any length of time, the trainer should emphasise strongly the potential dangers of over-training. As the identification

Table 4.3	Typical signs of over-training
Symptom category	**Symptom indication**
Movement/coordination	• Increased incidence of rhythm/movement problems. • Lack of prolonged concentration. • Reduced ability to correct movement errors.
Condition	• Decrease in endurance, strength speed, etc. • Can't cope with difficult situations such as competition. • Tries to deviate from set programme. • Negative attitude. Gives up easily.
Psychological	• Increased non-typical behaviour. • Anxiety, depression, lacks motivation. • Increased introvert behaviour.

SF-POMS QUESTIONNAIRE

Please read the statements below and give a score of 1–5

Statement	Score
I slept well last night	
I am looking forward to today's workout	
I am optimistic about future performance	
I feel vigorous and energetic	
I have little muscle soreness	
My appetite is great	
	Total =

Client name	Date
Mesocycle	Microcycle week
Yesterday's training intensity	
Previous score	Decision

Figure 4.8 Adapted Short-Form POMS Questionnaire (for a template visit: www.bloomsbury.com/9781408187234).

of over-training symptoms is difficult, even for those with experience, the trainer should consult with more qualified colleagues should they feel they lack the knowledge and experience in this particular area.

One of the reasons why the area of over-training is so controversial is that, even though the general consensus is that it does exist, there is no fool-proof diagnostic test. Anaemia or illness often present the same symptoms as over-training, so if suspected the trainer should make sure the client is seen by a health professional to rule out any illnesses. Some diagnostic tools are not easily available to the trainer, for example, hormonal and immune system functioning tests and ergometry work rate tests, but two tests that are relatively simple to administer, however, are psychological mood state and orthostatic heart rate response.

Mood state

There is an abundance of research available that suggests there is a link between mood changes and training status. To determine the mood state of an individual, there are many questionnaires generally available. One that is commonly used and appropriate for the health and fitness industry is the Profile of Mood States (POMS) Questionnaire, which was originally developed by McNair, Lorr and Droppleman in 1971 as an assessment method for people undergoing counselling or psychotherapy. As this was quite a lengthy questionnaire and not practical for use on a daily basis, the Short-Form POMS Questionnaire (SF-POMS) was subsequently developed by Curran and colleagues in 1995. Clients are recommended to use the SF-POMS Questionnaire on a daily basis or each time they see their trainer in order to try and determine signs of over-training.

It can be seen that the adapted short form includes options for the mesocycle and microcycle information to be added so that the trainer knows the stage of training at which the questionnaire was completed. The form also indicates the intensity of training on the previous day as it can have an effect on the outcome of the questionnaire over the days following the training. On completion of the questionnaire (normally done each morning) if the score is 20 or above, then the client is considered to be recovered enough to continue with the training program. If the score is below 20, then rest or an easy workout should be recommended (and recorded next to decision on the form) until the score rises above 20. When correctly used, the POMS Questionnaire has been shown to be effective in providing an early indication of over-training. Factors that should be considered, however, are that the answers given are very subjective and an individual may not be fully honest when filling out the questionnaire.

Orthostatic heart rate

Orthostasis is a debilitating disorder of the autonomic nervous system. In general terms it means that blood pressure and heart rate are strikingly different when lying down as opposed to standing up. For example, blood pressure and heart rate normally follow a similar pattern when standing upright from a lying or seated position but this pattern can change due to over-training.

Finnish researcher Heikki Rusko developed a protocol for testing orthostatic heart rate in order to identify potential over-training (and adaptation to training). The test involves measuring the heart rate of an individual when standing up from a lying position and for a short period of time afterwards. As the test is relatively easy to administer it can be done on a regular, if not daily, basis. The protocol (test procedure) is as follows:

Orthostatic Heart Rate Protocol:

1. Attach a heart rate monitor to the subject.
2. Get the subject to lie down in a comfortable supine (on the back) position.
3. Get the subject to relax until their heart rate has stabilised.
4. Once heart rate is stabilised start the stopwatch.
5. After 6 minutes record the subject's heart rate every 15 seconds.
6. After 8 minutes get the subject to stand up and stay standing for a further 2 minutes (still recording heart rate every 15 seconds).
7. At 10 minutes terminate the test.

Once the test has been completed the trainer could use a simple programme such as Excel to plot the results of the test. If a graph of the heart rate of the individual was plotted for the duration of the test, it would look something like that in figure 4.9.

A baseline test should be carried out at the start of a programme when the subject is well rested so that subsequent tests can be compared against it. Individuals who are not on the verge of over-training tend to have reasonably constant results day-to-day. The example in figure 4.9 shows a typical heart-rate response following a baseline test for a normal well-rested subject. If a subsequent test showed an elevated heart-rate average between 90 and 120 seconds after standing (i.e. 8–10+ beats above normal), this would be an indication of potential over-training (as indicated by the potential over-training line on the graph). Conversely, a heart rate trace dropping below the normal well-rested line may be an indication of positive adaptations to training (as indicated by the improving adaptation line).

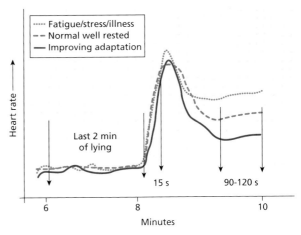

Figure 4.9 Typical heart rate response from lying to standing

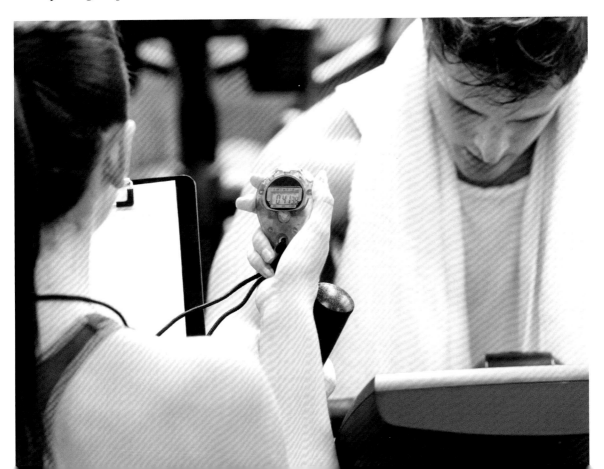

HOW TO TEACH AND ADAPT EXERCISES

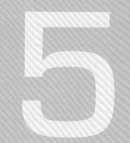

THE NOS LEVEL 3 PERSONAL TRAINER CRITERIA COVERED IN THIS CHAPTER ARE:

- The range of approved teaching and motivational styles you can use and how to vary these according to each client's response
- Why it is important to make sure your clients are properly prepared physically and psychologically before activity begins
- Why you should find out from your clients how they responded to previous physical activity and if anything has changed since then
- Why you should explain the objectives and activities you have planned to your clients
- Why your clients need to know the physical and technical demands of the activity and how this might affect their motivation
- Why it may be important to negotiate and agree changes to your plans with your clients
- Why and how any changes should be recorded
- Health, safety and emergency procedures and requirements and why your clients need to know these
- The importance of the warm-up and the range of warm-up activities you can use for the activities you are teaching
- How to choose warm-ups appropriate to different clients and conditions
- Why your clients should understand the purpose and value of the warm-up
- How to provide instructions, demonstrations and explanations clearly and effectively
- The correct positions for the exercises you are teaching
- How to adapt exercise positions as appropriate to individual clients and conditions
- The importance of demonstrating correct techniques and how to adopt appropriate teaching styles to make sure your clients apply techniques correctly
- How to modify the intensity of exercise to match each client's response to physical activity

- Why it is important to allow sufficient time for your clients to finish exercising and how you can adapt this to different levels of client needs and experience
- The purpose and value of cool-down activities and how to select these according to the type and intensity of physical exercise and client needs and condition
- Why your clients need to understand the value and purpose of cool-down
- Why your clients should be given the opportunity to ask questions, provide feedback and discuss their performance and how to make sure this happens
- Why your clients need to see their progress against objectives in terms of their overall goals and programme
- Why your clients need information about future activities, either supervised or not
- Procedures for dealing with equipment and the wider facility once the session is over

TEACHING EXERCISE SESSIONS

Although each client's goals will be different, a typical exercise session forming part of an overall exercise programme would normally include the following components (2, 3 and 4 recommended by the American College of Sports Medicine):

1. Introduction
2. Warm-up
3. Conditioning phase (including cardio, resistance and flexibility training)
4. Cool-down
5. In-session review

INTRODUCTION

There are several reasons why trainers should adopt the habit of having a brief pre-exercise session introduction, the main reason being that it helps to put the client at ease in what can often be a stressful situation for them. The trainer should always be on time for every session so that they are there to welcome the client. Thorough planning of the session will create an air of professionalism, which will help the client trust the trainer. This includes making sure all equipment needed for the session is available to avoid the session having to be adapted.

The introduction also gives the opportunity to discuss the previous session and how the client felt after that. It also gives the client an opportunity to raise any aspects of the session that they would like to change. And if the trainer has asked the client to provide any information – such as action plans or mood state forms – now is a good time to get that from them. Any changes to the programme should always be recorded for future discussion and reference.

To prepare the client mentally for the demands of the session, the trainer should give a brief overview of what to expect. This also gives the trainer the opportunity to link the activities of the session to the original client goals. Finally, at the end of the introduction the trainer should give a health and safety brief. This will normally cover the following areas:

- Emergency exit locations
- Fire procedures
- Water availability

- First aid person
- Telephone location

WARM-UP

Before exercising, it is essential that muscle and tendonous (fascia) tissue is fully warmed in order to reduce the potential for injury. Research generally agrees that the main way to prevent muscle injury is to raise the muscle temperature. Muscle is more elastic when warm and therefore will stretch easier without damage.

Regardless of the client and their ability, the intensity of the warm-up should increase gradually in order to avoid the build up of any lactic acid (a by-product of carbohydrate breakdown). It can be performed using cardiovascular equipment, such as a treadmill, rower, cycle or step machine or, if no equipment is available, through brisk walking or slow jogging. The type of exercise chosen for the warm-up depends on the equipment available, but should be specific to the goals of the client. For example, if the client has specific sporting goals such as fitness for rugby then the warm-up should mimic the movement of the sport (this is also referred to as a dynamic warm-up and examples can be found in *Teaching Exercise to Children* by Coulson) and be performed on grass if possible. Whatever the method chosen by the trainer the fundamental principles of a warm-up remain the same: the warm-up should aim to achieve a change in a number of physiological responses, in order that the body can operate safely and effectively.

Typical benefits include:

1. An increase in body temperature, specifically core muscle temperature
2. An increase in the elasticity of muscular and fascia tissue
3. A decreased risk of soft-tissue injury
4. Activation of the neuromuscular system
5. An increase in mental alertness.

In general a warm-up should take about 5–10 minutes and should facilitate the transition from rest to the level of exercise required in the main activity session that follows. Guidelines for a warm-up in terms of duration and intensity are:

- **Duration.** The ideal time period for a warm up depends on the environment and other factors but is usually no less than 5 minutes. If the weather or environment is hot, for instance, then the warm-up duration should be reduced. If the weather is cold, however, it makes sense to extend the warm-up period even if this encroaches on the time allowed for the main activity.
- **Intensity.** The warm-up should be designed to bring the entire muscular system into a state of readiness for exercise, as well as warming the muscles and fascia. As a general rule, the intensity of the warm-up should progressively increase with a view to end at the level that the main activity intends to start.

COOL-DOWN

The cool-down is sometimes referred to as a 'warm-down' and these two terms can be used interchangeably. As the cool-down follows the main activity of the session, clients need to take time to gradually reduce their heart rate and blood pressure to near resting levels. As a general guide, the intensity levels of the exercise should be reduced gradually throughout the cool-down until the heart rate is below 100 bpm. The ACSM recommends a period of approximately

5–10 minutes for this part of the exercise session. Clients can use the same type of cardiovascular equipment used in the warm-up to achieve this, but at a level that gradually reduces in intensity. In general terms, the cool-down should help to:

1. Disperse lactic acid
2. Prevent blood pooling
3. Return the body systems to normal levels
4. Assist in maintaining venous return
5. Reduce the potential for hypotension and dizziness
6. Help to dissipate body heat.

Research has shown that performing a cool-down can help reduce the 'stiff' feeling that can occur in the days following intense exercise activities. Another benefit is that it can help maintain blood circulation after exercise. In simple terms, when exercise comes to an abrupt stop, the heart continues to beat at a fast rate and therefore pumps a lot of blood which builds up in the lower legs (this is known as blood pooling). This happens because muscular contraction, as a result of moving around, is one of the main mechanisms responsible for helping blood get back to the heart; a process known as venous return. Moving around and gradually reducing the heart rate has been shown to prevent this from happening. General guidelines in terms of duration and intensity are:

- **Duration.** The cool-down can be of varying duration depending on the environment, intensity level of the main activity and fitness level of the client. For instance, cool-downs in warmer environments would be longer than those in colder environments. Also, if the main

activity component was high intensity, then the cool-down should be longer. If the main activity was low intensity, then the cool-down could be done quickly. Trainers should also consider that fitter clients will recover quicker than less fit clients. As a guide the cool-down would be between 5 to 10 minutes, which should be included as part of the session.

- **Intensity.** The whole point of doing the cool-down is to try and gradually reduce the heart rate levels so that the heart is not pumping lots of blood around the body. The cool-down intensity should start from the point at the end of the main activity component and gradually reduce in intensity until clients have recovered to near resting levels.

CONDITIONING PHASE

Sometimes referred to as the main activity, the conditioning phase is the part of the session that focuses on the improvement of the client's health and fitness components. This phase would normally include cardiovascular, resistance and flexibility training, unless the trainer had designed a split programme in which only certain components are addressed. Trainers may choose to perform the cool-down component prior to the flexibility exercises (static stretches are recommended at this point) depending on the nature of the particular session. There is no recommended duration for the conditioning phase as this would be goal specific and affected by many variables such as time availability of the client and any health conditions they may have.

IN-SESSION REVIEW

A brief review should be built in to every exercise session as this allows the client to discuss any important aspects of the session while it is still fresh in their mind. The best time to do this would be at the end of the session. Within this review trainers should point out any progression that has been made and how this links to goals that have been set. It also allows the trainer to reinforce any instructions or advice that they have given the client during their session. This is important as clients may have unsupervised sessions before their next meeting with their trainer. Finally, the review should always include a quick 'housekeeping' check to make sure that any equipment that was used had been returned to its correct stowage so that there are no potential hazards for other users (even though this should have been done on an on-going basis during the session).

All trainers should aim to give their clients value for money. Therefore, the balance of instruction, exercise and discussion should be tailored to each client. Most clients prefer to be involved in as much exercise as possible; therefore, limit the amount of discussion for these clients and try to drip-feed information during the session and, if possible, back this up with written materials, such as hand-outs or pamphlets.

INDUCTION

Induction is a term that is used before a client begins an exercise programme. It's an opportunity for the trainer to show the client how the equipment works and what their exercise session will involve. As well as explaining how to operate any equipment, the induction should take the client through each component of the exercise session in turn (warm-up, cardio, cool-down, resistance and flexibility) to make sure they understand and practise each component. It is important that trainers brief clients on the importance of each component as they progress through the induction session. Another purpose of the induction is to identify client training intensities in relation to cardiovascular and resistance equipment settings – i.e. setting levels and speeds on cardiovascular equipment and weight used on resistance machines or free-weights.

There are no specific guidelines relating to client induction procedures. However, common guidelines can be adapted to suit the personal trainer. These guidelines relate to a client induction for the cardiovascular, resistance and flexibility components of the session to be performed.

WARM-UP, CARDIO AND COOL-DOWN INDUCTION

The facility in which the trainer is working will determine the type of cardiovascular exercise prescribed. The session may not require the use of cardiovascular machines but if it does, trainers are advised to familiarise themselves with the machines prior to inducting clients.

Before clients begin a programme of exercise, they need to be given an induction relating to their exercise programme. Following an explanation of the controls of any cardiovascular machines being used, the trainer should take the client through their session in order to establish cardiovascular intensity levels for the warm-up, main activity and cool-down. In terms of the warm-up, the trainer may choose to incorporate a dynamic flexibility routine, utilise a range of cardiovascular machines or just employ light jogging with a steady increase in intensity. Whatever method chosen and for the purpose of consistency of delivery, it is advisable to use a logical approach such as an adaptation of the IDEA method:

I Introduce the exercise

D Demonstrate the correct technique

E Evaluate the exercise using minimal coaching points

A Assess (and record) the intensity level suitable for the particular component.

I Introduce the exercise. State the name of the exercise and its purpose. Repetition of this information should help the client remember it so that, when they work on their own, sessions can be discussed with the trainer without having to describe each exercise.

D Demonstrate the correct technique. It is important that trainers use correct technique when demonstrating so that the client does not copy bad technique. As a visual demonstration can provide a great deal of information, verbal information can be kept to a minimum. Even though a vast range of cardiovascular training equipment is available, there are many common guidelines that can be employed when using the equipment (see appendix 3).

E Evaluate the exercise using minimal coaching points. Following the demonstration by the trainer, the client should perform the exercise. When the client is performing the exercise, the trainer should talk them through the performance and technique. The trainer should let the client know how to carry out the exercise safely and effectively.

A Assess (and record) the intensity level. The trainer should aim to identify the suitable training intensity for each component. If cardiovascular equipment is being used, then information can be easily gathered from the actual machine in terms of speed, RPM, stroke rate, etc. However, if no cardiovascular equipment is being used the trainer will need to gauge the intensity level of each component.

Monitoring cardiovascular intensity

During a warm-up, cardio activity or cool-down, the intensity of the exercise should be controlled so that it is suitable for the goals of the individual client. For example, if the goal of a client is to increase aerobic capacity, it is important that the training intensity remains at the appropriate level. Several methods can be used to prescribe and monitor cardiovascular exercise intensity including heart rate, self-perception (rate of perceived exertion) and communication skills (the talk test).

Heart rate

One of the most common methods of monitoring cardiovascular intensity is the heart rate method. Before monitoring the heart rate during each component, the trainer should have calculated the heart rate of the client at the relevant percentage of maximum (written as %HRM) for each component. There are two steps to convert the chosen percentage of heart rate maximum into beats per minute. First, the maximum heart rate of the client needs to be found; second, the heart rate at the required percentage of this maximum needs to be calculated.

Step 1: Calculating the maximum heart rate of an individual.

As maximum graded heart rate tests are not suitable for all clients, a predicted method should be used such as the formula:

- Maximum Heart Rate = 220 − age

For example, a 23-year-old person would have a predicted maximum heart rate of 197bpm (220–23 = 197) and a 45-year-old person would have a predicted maximum heart rate of 175bpm (220–45). Even though there are errors associated with this method of estimating maximum heart rate (there can be an error of plus or minus 12bpm using this method), it is commonly used throughout the health and fitness industry.

Step 2: Calculating heart rate at the chosen percentage of the maximum heart rate.

Once the maximum heart rate has been established, the percentage of maximum heart rate that is required for the client in beats per minute (bpm) can be calculated: the maximum heart rate for the client is multiplied by the chosen percentage. For example, a 32-year-old client needs to perform exercise at 70–80 per cent of maximum heart rate (the aerobic zone). The trainer should calculate the client's training intensity heart rates at 70 and 80 per cent of maximum as follows:

1. Predicted maximum heart rate for the individual is 220–age (32) = 188 bpm
2. 70 per cent of maximum (188 bpm) = 188/100 × 70 = 131 bpm
3. 80 per cent of maximum (188 bpm) = (188/100 × 80) = 150 bpm

NB: Round the answer to the nearest whole number.

Therefore, in order to exercise at the desired intensity, the client would need to keep their heart rate between 131bpm and 150bpm. Over a period of time, if the client could maintain this heart rate but at an increased speed, this would indicate they were becoming fitter.

Tip

There are other methods of predicting maximum heart rate (see appendix 4).

Rate of perceived exertion (RPE)

Another method of setting and monitoring the appropriate exercise intensity for a client is to use the rate of perceived exertion (RPE) scale (see figure 5.1), first introduced by Dr Gunnar Borg and known as the Borg scale. The RPE scale is a method of measuring the subjective feelings of an individual during exercise. Perception of the level of difficulty during cardiovascular exercise has been found to correlate very strongly with heart rate.

Two different scales are commonly used: the 6–20 scale and the revised 0–10+ scale, also known as the category ratio or CR-10 scale. Essentially, a client is shown the scale during exercise and asked how he or she feels compared to the words on the scale. This perception is then used to estimate either the percentage of heart rate maximum or the heart rate. For example, if the client states that the exercise feels 'somewhat hard', this equates to level 13 on the 6–20 scale, which corresponds to approximately 130bpm or 75 per cent of MHR.

RATE OF PERCEIVED EXERTION (BORG) SCALE

6–20 scale	0–10 scale	Estimate of %MHR
6	0 Nothing at all	
7 Very, very light	0.3	
8	0.5 Extremely weak	50%
9 very light	0.7	55%
10	1 Very weak	60%
11 Fairly light	1.5	65%
12	2 Weak	70%
13 Somewhat hard	2.5	75%
14	3 Moderate	80%
15 Hard	4	85%
16	5 Strong	88%
17 Very hard	6	92%
18	7 Very strong	96%
19 Very, very hard	8	98%
20	9	100%
	10 Extremely strong	
	11	
	Absolute maximum	

Figure 5.1 Borg RPE scales correlated to %HRM (adapted from *ACSM Guidelines for Exercise Testing and Prescription*. Lippincott, Williams and Wilkins, 2006)

Depending on the goals of the client, the trainer can recommend an RPE level at which to exercise without the need to monitor heart rate. Even though the subjective perception of exercise intensity correlates well with heart rate, it is important to note that various individuals carrying out exactly the same exercise session might report different levels of RPE. There are many factors that could affect this perception rating, such as fitness levels, exercise familiarity and illness.

Talk test

Although the talk test is not a particularly scientific method of determining cardiovascular exercise intensity, it can be used as an alternative to heart rate or RPE and it's an easy one to carry out. The talk test is simply a matter of talking to the client during exercise and gauging the level of intensity from the response. If the client is able to carry out a normal conversation, this usually indicates that he or she is exercising aerobically. If the client becomes breathless and has difficulty maintaining a normal conversation, this usually means he or she is exercising anaerobically. The trainer can then adjust the level of intensity accordingly.

RESISTANCE INDUCTION

Most beginners to resistance training are unfamiliar with the operation of body-weight exercises, resistance machines or free weights. It is therefore important to give clear explanations of how to perform body-weight exercise or operate resistance machines before the client begins an exercise programme. As with the cardio induction, the trainer usually takes the client through their resistance training session in order to establish intensity levels. There are many methods of inducting individuals in relation to resistance training, depending on the individual trainer's preference. However, in order to be consistent in the delivery, it is advisable to use a logical approach such as the NAMSIT method:

N Name the machine or body-weight exercise
A Area of the body working
M Muscle group name
S Silent demonstration
I Instruct client
T Training intensity

N **Name the machine or body-weight exercise.** When introducing the client to the exercise it is important to state the name of the exercise that they are going to perform. For example: 'this machine is called the chest press' or 'this exercise is called a full press up'.

A **Area of the body working.** It is also useful to tell the client which area of the body the exercise will affect. The trainer should also indicate this using their hand as a visual cue.

M **Muscle group name.** Try to empower the client to learn muscle group names by stating them when showing which area the exercise affects.

S **Silent demonstration.** It is important that trainers use good technique when demonstrating to prevent the individual picking up bad habits. As with all components, the visual demonstration for resistance exercises will provide a lot of information so supplementary verbal information should be kept to a minimum.

I **Instruct client.** Get the client to perform the exercise. During the exercise the trainer should comment on their client's performance and technique. At this point the trainer should tell the client how to carry out the exercise safely and effectively.

T **Training intensity.** The trainer should then identify the intensity required for each resistance exercise. If resistance equipment is being used, information can be easily gathered. However, if no equipment is being used, the trainer will need to gauge the intensity level.

Monitoring resistance intensity

When prescribing and monitoring the intensity of a resistance exercise, the trainer should use a system known as 'repetition maximum' or RM. The maximum weight a client can lift for one repetition is known as their '1RM'. It follows that a multiple of the repetition maximum, such as 10RM or 15RM, is the maximum weight the individual can lift 10 or 15 times respectively. The ACSM guidelines for strength and endurance are given in multiples of RM. For example, in order to gain strength it is recommended that an individual performs resistance exercise using weights within the range of 8–12RM, and to improve endurance using weights within the range of 10–15RM. When trying to establish the amount of weight a client can lift for a specific number of repetitions (repetition maximum), a standardised procedure should be used. This process should then be done for all of the exercises in the resistance training component.

1. Select a load that is about 50% of the client's chosen RM.
2. Get the client to perform 5–10 repetitions (use as a warm-up).
3. Get feedback from the client as to the difficulty level.
4. Adjust the weight but only increase by small increments.
5. After a short rest (1 minute) get the client to perform a few repetitions and repeat steps 3 and 4 until the client fails to do one more repetition than the chosen RM.

Tip
Make sure enough rest is given between efforts.

Assuming that the number of repetitions remains the same, when the client is capable of comfortably performing repetitions the weight can be increased by a small amount. If the client cannot perform the number of repetitions at the increased weight, he or she must revert to the original weight. This type of in-built progression is easy to implement and the trainer should empower the client to take control of monitoring their own progression.

FLEXIBILITY INDUCTION

It is common for static stretches to be done following the cool-down as the heart rate should be at near resting levels and connective tissue fully warmed. As with any other part of the induction it is important that the trainer provides a technically correct demonstration of all the stretches included in the exercise programme. If in a gym environment, the trainer should utilise a matted area for stretching. If the session is outdoors, then the trainer should make sure that they have a stretch mat available otherwise standing stretches may be the only option. When mats are available it is logical to start with standing stretches and then progress to seated stretches in order to progressively decrease the heart rate. Trainers could also use the NAMSIT method for stretches. For example, once the trainer has named the stretch and the area it affects they can demonstrate the stretch then get the client to perform it. The trainer should then give feedback about the client's technique and give instructions about the intensity and duration of the stretch.

// INSTRUCTING

6

THE NOS LEVEL 3 PERSONAL TRAINER CRITERIA COVERED IN THIS CHAPTER ARE:

- Why it is important to make sure your clients understand your instructions, demonstrations and explanations
- The importance of non-verbal communication and body language
- The communication skills needed to assist clients with motivation:
  - how to ask open-ended questions
  - active listening skills
  - methods of gathering personal information
  - appropriate questioning techniques
  - interpreting client responses including body language and other forms of behaviour especially when undertaking physical activity
  - means of summarising gathered information
- How to adapt communication to meet each client's needs
- The importance of matching teaching and learning styles to maximise clients' progress and motivation
- Why a balance of instruction, exercise and discussion is necessary
- How to utilise verbal and non-verbal communication techniques
- The importance of careful and thorough planning and preparation before exercise
- Methods you can use to get structured feedback from clients
- Why structured feedback is important
- How to analyse information and client feedback
- Why it is important to discuss preliminary conclusions with the client
- Why the clients' views are important

Autocratic		Democratic	
Telling	**Selling**	**Sharing**	**Allowing**
Trainer decides on what is to be done	Trainer decides what is to be done	Trainer outlines session to the clients	Trainer outlines the session to the clients
Clients not involved in any decisions	Trainer explains objectives	Trainer invites ideas from the clients	Trainer defines conditions
Trainer defines what and how to do it	Clients encouraged to question and confirm understanding	Trainer makes decisions based on clients' suggestions	Clients explore possible ideas.
Clients told the exercises	Trainer defines what and how to do it	Trainer defines what and how to do it	Clients make the decision
	Trainer explains the object of the session and purpose of each exercise	Trainer identifies a session outline	Clients define what and how to do it
	Clients ask questions	Clients identify possible exercises for the session	Trainer identifies a session
		Trainer selects from the suggestions	Trainer defines conditions of the session
			Clients identify exercises for the session that meet the instructor's conditions

Figure 6.1 Autocratic and democratic instructing styles and their sub-types

INSTRUCTING

There are many ways in which people instruct but perhaps the two most common styles are those of 'autocratic' (do as I say) and 'democratic' (clients help in decision making). The autocratic style can be further split into two types, that of 'telling' and 'selling' and the democratic style into 'sharing' and 'allowing'. Figure 6.1 gives a visual overview of both styles and their respective types.

Trainers do not usually use only one style throughout a session but often use a variety of styles depending on the situation and the client they are instructing at that particular time. It is important that trainers be aware of client responses to various methods and attempt to match the instruction style to what best suits the client. This will maximise the client's progress and motivation.

Other styles of instructing include the 'command' and 'reciprocal' style.

- **Command style.** Similar to the autocratic telling style, the command style is when there is direct instruction and the trainer makes all the decisions for the clients to follow. This style assumes that the trainer knows what they are talking about so the client listens.

INSTRUCTING

- **Reciprocal style** (also known as cooperative style). Similar to the democratic style, the reciprocal style is where the client takes some responsibility for their own development, although this is monitored and guided by the trainer. There are two different methods a trainer can adopt under the banner of reciprocal style. 'Problem solving', in which the client solves problems set by the trainer and 'guided discovery' in which the client has freedom to explore various ideas or options. These two methods are often used with clients who are familiar with gym training. With problem solving, for example, a client may express the wish of increasing muscle bulk but doesn't think they eat enough protein in their diet. The trainer could then challenge the client to estimate their protein requirement and research what forms of protein would be appropriate for them. As a guided discovery method the trainer could allow a degree of freedom in which to test out the impact of various protein intakes over a period of time in order to find the best approach that suited the client.

Those new to instructing tend to adopt the command style as they can just dictate and avoid questions until they feel they are sufficiently knowledgeable. Unfortunately the command style usually only favours the highly motivated athlete and doesn't really suit the majority of clients. The reciprocal style still allows the trainer to guide and make decisions but it is up to the trainer to make it look as though the client has had a say in the decision-making process. For instance, in the previous example, the trainer could say, 'have you thought about protein supplementation?', which might encourage a favourable response by the client who might have thought it was a good idea but just needed affirmation. This way the client might think it was originally their idea.

One of the main purposes of instructing is to empower the client to perform exercises safely following guidance and demonstration by the trainer. The ability to do this requires specific skills on the part of the trainer such as communication, observation, correction and feedback. Skills such as these are often considered crucial to the successful retention of clients.

COMMUNICATION

There are three methods of communication that the trainer can use, verbal (with an emphasis on speaking), para-verbal (through voice tone and stress on words) and non-verbal (by the use of gestures).

VERBAL COMMUNICATION

Humans are not good at retaining much verbal information so it is wise not to give too many verbal instructions. It is also important for the trainer to try and talk in a simple and clear way so that clients are not confused and suffer from information overload. In order to demonstrate this, try the activity in figure 6.2.

It is easy to assume that verbal communication is related only to speaking. But listening is also an important facet of verbal communication.

Listening skills

Most people 'hear' but don't 'listen'. For example, have you ever met anyone for the first time and within a few minutes you can't remember their name? One of the reasons for this is that individuals often place more importance on

TRY THIS

You will need pens and paper enough for a small group of people.

What to do   Give the group a pen and paper. Read out a 7-digit number, get the group to wait for 5 seconds then ask them to write down the number (they have to remember it obviously). Do this again but use an 8-digit number and ask them to write it down after a 5-second wait. You should find that most of them would have written the 7-digit number down correctly but didn't cope with the 8-digit number.

Why does   This is a phenomenon called 'chunking'. Very simply, if the brain thinks it will
it happen?   be overloaded it will tend only to remember the first and last bits of a piece of information.

Figure 6.2 Example of information overload

what they have to say than rather than on what others have to say. Generally speaking, there are two types of listening, that of passive and active listening.

- **Passive listening.** This can be described as listening without any kind of response. Passive listening is appropriate in some situations such as watching a movie or listening to music, but in an instructing situation the speaker (this could be the trainer or the client) would not know that the listener has understood what was said if there was no response.
- **Active listening.** This type of listening requires a response to show understanding. In active listening, the trainer might have to respond to general statements or questions from clients depending on the context or the situation. For example, scenario 1 and scenario 2 give examples of a client asking a typical question and also making a typical statement. The scenarios give just one of many possible trainers' responses.

Scenario 1. *'Do you think I will have a good session today?'*
This seems like a fairly harmless question but clients often ask this because they need reinforcement and encouragement due to low confidence and a fear of failure. One way the trainer could respond is by saying 'As long as you try your best then I will be really happy'. In this way the trainer is showing understanding of the question but reinforcing that not doing as well is fine because it is the effort and participation that is important.

Scenario 2. *'I think that I did really well today'.*
The trainer must consider the response carefully. For instance, the client may not have done well so the trainer may need to make the client aware of this. In this scenario the trainer could ask another question such as 'Did you think all of the session was good, or were there things you think you could improve?'

This would show that the trainer listened and would open up a debate to help point out areas for improvement. If the client did do well, in most cases they still need encouragement. In this scenario the trainer could say 'you did well today but tell me, is there anything you want to improve on for next time?' Again this shows understanding but challenges the client to always try harder.

As can be seen from both scenarios, responding to a client's statement or question is not always as straightforward as it might seem. Often there is an underlying message that the client is trying to communicate. Experience is invaluable in these cases as each scenario can have many outcomes depending on each response of both the client and the trainer.

PARA-VERBAL COMMUNICATION

This type of communication is related to the use of words and the structure of sentences. Placing stress on different words in a sentence can change the meaning of the sentence. Emotion is often reflected in para-verbal communication as clients will often pick up on excitement and enthusiasm but care must be taken as clients could also pick up on sadness and boredom.

NON-VERBAL COMMUNICATION

To communicate non-verbally just means getting a point across without speaking. Over 70% of communication is done through non-verbal means. Also known as 'body language', this can

Table 6.1	Categories of non-verbal communication
Sub-Category	**Strategies**
Role Model	The way in which you look and dress can often influence clients. If you do not look after yourself physically, it will give an indication to the client that you are not bothered about fitness. Also if you do not dress appropriately this could have an effect on clients as well.
Body Position	The way you position yourself with clients is very important. Don't get too close (in their 'personal space') as it could intimidate them. Also do not turn your back as this is often construed as having been given the 'cold shoulder'.
Body Movements	Simple gestures with the eyes, hands, head, etc., can be very effective. For example, a tilt of the head to the side with furrowed eyebrows can easily say 'why did you do that?'
Voice	You will often have heard the saying 'it's not what you say but how you say it'. People easily pick up on how we say things so avoid sarcasm. You also need to speak with enough volume to be heard but speak slowly and try to articulate so there is no confusion with translation.

be used by the trainer to communicate messages to the client or as a means of interpreting client responses, especially when undertaking physical activity. There are various sub-categories of non-verbal communication and table 6.1 gives a description of just some of the strategies used to communicate certain messages to the client.

Whatever method of communication is being used, the trainer should always encourage clients to ask questions. It is also useful for the trainer to ask the client if they have understood the instructions, again to avoid any misunderstanding. This should help give the trainer an understanding of how instructions are being perceived so that they can modify or adapt their communication method should it be required.

OBSERVATION

During all supervised sessions the trainer needs to observe the client, but there are also times when the client need to observe the trainer. In terms of the trainer observing the client, this can be split into three main areas: safety, performance and reinforcement.

Safety

One of the most important objectives of a training session is to maintain the safety of the client. There are many potential hazards and dangers in an exercise environment and it is crucial that the trainer is being attentive at all times. It is best to be positioned (as much as is possible) where the trainer can see the face of the client so that they can monitor the client for signs of any undue distress in order that the exercise can be stopped as soon as possible if necessary.

Performance

During all exercises the trainer needs to constantly monitor the performance of the client. One reason for this is that facial expressions and appearance can often indicate the intensity level of the particular exercise. Another reason is that the trainer needs to ensure good technique. It may be necessary to walk around the client in order to view how different body segments are positioned either statically or in motion.

Reinforcement

When a client is performing an exercise (especially a resistance exercise) it is useful for the trainer to reinforce correct movement. This can be done using the 'mirroring' technique where the trainer stands in front (or in the best position to be seen) of the client and performs the exercise being done so that the client can mirror the action. This is a technique can also be used to set the pace of an exercise when the client is going too fast.

Correction

Well-executed demonstrations often reduce the need for correction, but correction of technique is usually required especially in the early stages of an exercise programme for those clients with little or no previous exercise experience. Once the trainer has ensured that the exercise is being carried out safely it is then their role to assess technique and adjust if necessary. In a one-to-one situation this is relatively straightforward as the mirroring technique could be used with a few verbal comments if needed. In a group situation, however, the approach is slightly different in order to avoid singling out any individual. The method here is called the GET approach, as shown in figure 6.3.

GENERAL
Make the feedback comment
to the whole group without
looking at any individual

⬇

EYE CONTACT
Repeat the comment but
make eye contact with the
individual

⬇

TALK
Speak discreetly to the
individual/s

Figure 6.3 The GET approach

If a correction is needed to an individual in a group (but there is no safety issue), the trainer should make a general (G) comment to the whole group without looking at just the individual that the comment is directed at. For example, 'make sure you keep neutral spine and strong core throughout the full range of the squat'. If the individual/s did not respond to this, then the trainer should repeat the comment but this time making eye contact with the individual/s (E) without being too obvious. If there is no response in terms of improving technique, the trainer should talk (T) directly to the individual concerned and instruct them on a one-to-one basis.

FEEDBACK

The client gets two forms of feedback – from external sources, known as 'extrinsic feedback' and from internal

sources known as 'intrinsic feedback'. Figure 6.4 gives some examples of both extrinsic and intrinsic feedback sources.

- **Extrinsic feedback.** Sources of extrinsic feedback include the client getting information about the performance from other people, such as the trainer. For example, the trainer could make the comment about the running style of the client. There can be clashes with feedback – if the client takes part in sports or events, teammates and friends might also give feedback, which may be detrimental to the goals of the client. The client should be made aware of this.
- **Intrinsic feedback.** Intrinsic feedback is related to the feelings and senses of the client during performance. An example of this could be when a client is performing a stretch and the trainer is asking them to feel and comment on the tightness in the relevant muscle.

Giving feedback to the client can take place both during the performance and afterwards. In both cases the feedback should be positive but, during the performance, should be limited to minor correction points and regular praise, which helps the client's motivation.

Most clients need motivation at some point, which often works well when it comes from

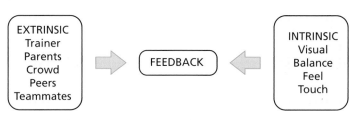

EXTRINSIC
Trainer
Parents
Crowd
Peers
Teammates

➡ FEEDBACK ⬅

INTRINSIC
Visual
Balance
Feel
Touch

Figure 6.4 Types and examples of feedback

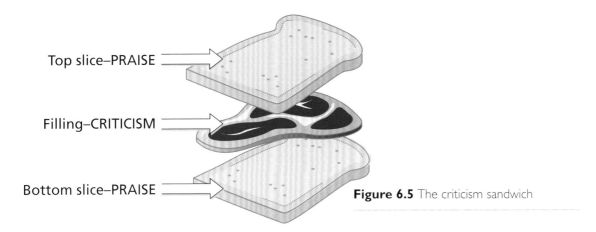

Top slice–PRAISE

Filling–CRITICISM

Bottom slice–PRAISE

Figure 6.5 The criticism sandwich

an external source such as the trainer. Positive comments and reminders of goals should always be used, rather than negative comments. At the end of the session, the feedback can be more explicit and linked to the client goals.

The criticism sandwich

When giving feedback to a client there is often a concern that any correction points may be perceived as criticism. It can be useful to compliment the correction points with positive praise. This is known as the 'criticism sandwich' as shown in figure 6.5. For example, the trainer may start with the positive statement 'you tried really hard today' followed by 'but I really need you to focus on running on your mid-foot' and end with another positive statement 'however, you are ahead of your short-term goal so I am very pleased'.

As well as the client getting feedback from various sources, the trainer also needs to get feedback from the client on a regular basis in relation to their perception of the performance. This is crucial for many reasons, such as adjusting the level of intensity of the exercise or changing an exercise for future sessions because the client doesn't like or enjoy that exercise. The trainer needs to do this

as often as possible without being too repetitious in terms of the questioning. For example, if the trainer needs to know how the client is coping with the speed during a 20-minute run, then the question can be phrased in several ways such as:

* Are you feeling ok at this level?
* Do you think you can go any faster?
* Do you need to slow down at all?
* How would you judge the RPE at the moment?
* Does this pace suit you?
* Can you continue at this pace for the rest of the duration?

Questions where the response is limited to one or two word answers are known as 'closed questions' as in the examples above. This is appropriate while clients are exercising whereas 'open-ended' questions are more appropriate when the client is not exercising (during rest or break periods) in order to elicit a more detailed response. For example, asking the question 'what do you think about the treadmill session you did today?' gives the client the opportunity to express their views in full. Both types of question are important as long as they are used in the correct context at the appropriate time.

83

REVIEW AND ADAPT PROGRAMMES

THE NOS LEVEL 3 PERSONAL TRAINER CRITERIA COVERED IN THIS CHAPTER ARE:

- How to communicate information to your clients and provide effective feedback
- Why it is important to encourage your clients to give their views
- How to analyse, monitor and record each client's progress
- Why it is important to agree changes with your clients
- Why it is important to communicate progress and changes to those involved
- Why it is important to keep accurate records of changes and the reasons for change
- How the principles of training can be used to adapt the programme where goals are not being achieved or new goals have been identified
- How to review short- medium- and long-term goals with your clients, taking into account any changes in circumstances
- How to communicate adaptations to your clients and other professionals
- When it may be necessary to adapt planned exercises to meet clients' needs and how to do so
- How to identify specific objectives from the overall programme goals
- Why it is important to evaluate progressive physical activity programmes
- The principles of evaluation in the context of physical activity
- What information is needed to evaluate physical activity programmes
- Methods you can use to collect the required information
- Why it is important to evaluate all stages and components of the programme
- Methods you can use to organise information so that you can analyse it

PROGRAMME MANAGEMENT

Once a programme of exercise has been designed for a client (and prior to an induction) it is important that all the necessary information is then put together and presented to the client in a manner that they fully understand and can easily follow. This should take place at an initial client review meeting so that the designed programme can be agreed and a schedule of follow-up review meetings can be drawn up.

During the initial review clients should be given copies of the weekly session profile (see example on page 58) so that they have a simple visual overview of how the exercise sessions fit into their personal weekly schedule. Clients will also need specific information relating to each individual session and the amount of information required will vary depending on the experience of the client. For those clients who have had previous experience of training programmes the information on the microcycle record sheets (see pages 59–61) will probably be sufficient. There will be those clients, however, who have little or no previous experience of training programmes, and then a more detailed presentation of information is be required. Figures 7.1 and 7.2 are examples of an individual session card (front and back) that can be used by the trainer for this particular purpose.

The trainer should always discuss the full details of the exercise programme with the client, explaining how the prescribed exercises were developed based on individual goals and how each component of fitness was built into the programme. At the end of the client review session the trainer should allow the client to take away all relevant information so that they have the opportunity to absorb it and to question and clarify any aspects that they are unsure about. It is important that clients are given this opportunity and encouraged to express their opinions otherwise it could have a potential negative effect to their adherence to the programme.

The amount of information that is given to each client will differ depending on the client and the programme designed. If a session card, such as that in figures 7.1 & 7.2, is used, the type of information relating to actual speeds, levels, weight, etc., can be gathered during the induction session and recorded on the card for subsequent sessions. It is also useful to agree and record on the session card a follow-up review date (or series of dates) so that the trainer and client can discuss any progress that might need to be made.

REVIEWS/RE-TESTS

Any review dates can be discussed and agreed with the client whenever a change is made to the programme or alternatively at the end of each mesocycle, whichever comes first. It is important to emphasise to the client that follow-up review meetings are fundamental to the success of any exercise programme as there are many circumstances that can easily affect health and fitness components. As a result it is vital to continually monitor circumstances with a view to prioritising certain components in order to achieve specific goals. The session card can also include the date

> **Tip**
>
> It would be useful for the trainer to print these out on card so that it is double-sided with a back and front. The client could then keep the session card with them during sessions as a quick reference guide.

SESSION CARD – FRONT

Client name	Week	Date	To
Programme review date	Re-test date	Contact	

WARM-UP:

Timing	Exercise & machine used	Level/Speed: Gradient: RPM or SPM:	Teaching / coaching points	RPE	Alternative and progression
4-5 mins	Rowing Machine	24-28	Make sure foot straps are correct and set the lowest level.	2-5	Cycle or cross trainer. No progression at this stage.

MAIN CARDIO AND COOL-DOWN:

20 mins	Treadmill	Speed 8kph	Reinforce the machine operation. Encourage running on the balls of the feet, keep shoulders relaxed and maintain neutral spine. Try to maintain a level where you can talk but not comfortably. Start at RPE level 5 and gradually increase to level 8 within 4 minutes.	5-8	When comfortable the speed can be adjusted to suit the RPE level. Increase the gradient 1% every 4 weeks (up to 3%).
4-5 mins	Cycle	RPM of 70-60 Level 4-1	Gradually decrease the RPM from 70 down to 60 and the level from 4 down to 1. Aim to get heart rate down to below 100bpm.	8-3	Cross trainer or walk on treadmill.

RESISTANCE:

Exercise/machine	RM/weight	Teaching / coaching points	Rest	Alternative and progression
Bent Over Row	14, 14, 12–60kg	Keep neutral spine and tension in TA.	1 min between sets	Db exercises should be free. Use tricep push down if cable busy. Increase the weight by the smallest amount when you can do more than 14 reps with the 14RM weight (same for 12 and 16RM).
Db Chest Press	14, 14, 12–24kg	Limit decent so upper arm parallel with floor.		
Db Shoulder Press	14, 14, 12–16kg	Dbs no lower than shoulder level.		
Tricep Over Head (Double)	12, 10, 10–20kg	Keep forearm in swimming position.		
Db Bicep Curl (Single)	14, 14, 12–12kg	Avoid twisting motion.		
Internal/External Rotation	16, 16, 14–15kg	Lie on side using Db or use cable in standing position (out to in and in to out).		

Figure 7.1 Individual session card (front) (for a blank template visit: www.bloomsbury.com/9781408187234).

RESISTANCE CONT'D:

Exercise/machine	RM	Teaching / coaching points.	Rest	Alternative and progression
Alternating: Squat	12, 10, 10, 12, 12 (70kg) 5 sets of 40 metres	Full ROM. Contract TA.	2 min between sets	• Swiss ball squat against wall, use dumbbells in each hand for added resistance • Rear, walking or side lunges can also be an effective way of changing the workout. • Unilateral leg press, using one leg at a time instead of two to press weight.
Bounding		Quick land-to-take-off phase.		
Alternating: Split Squat	12, 10, 10, 12, 12 (60kg) 5 sets (6)	Set on one leg then set on the other.		
Box Jump		Full foot contact on box.		

CORE STABILITY:

Exercise/machine	RM	Teaching / coaching points.	Rest	Alternative and progression
Supine Foot Slide Supine Knee Rolls	3 sets of 5 slides each leg and rolls.	Maintain natural curve in lumbar spine. Try to keep pelvis stable.	1 min between sets	All stability exercises to be done to fatigue or loss of form.
Superman	Hold for 10–15 seconds 5 times.	Hold the start position of neutral spine throughout and head facing floor.		

FLEXIBILITY:

Exercise/machine	RM	Teaching / coaching points.	Rest	Alternative and progression
Pectorals And Deltoids	15 seconds × 3	Clasp hands behind back and straighten arms, raise arms for more tension and keep back neutral.	N/A	• No progression at this time. • Quad stretch can be done in side-lying or standing position. • Hamstring stretch can be done standing with outstretched leg on low bench.
General Back/Shoulder	15 seconds × 3	Clasp hands in front of body, straighten arms away from body and push shoulder blades forward.		
Quadriceps	15 seconds × 3	Bring foot up towards bottom keeping knees together and maintain neutral back.		
Hamstrings	15 seconds × 3	Seated with back upright. One leg straight lean forward towards toes.		

Figure 7.2 Individual session card (back) (for a blank template visit: www.bloomsbury.com/9781408187234).

Client name   Week   Date   to

MESOCYCLE GOALS:

Baseline testing before week 1. Introduce core stabilisation and flexibility exercises. Introduce cardio training (aerobic). Assess resistance training ability and start with light weights to develop ligament strength.

PREVIOUS TEST RESULTS:

VO$_2$max: 56mlO2/kg/min	OBLA: 15km/hr	Chest press: 105kg	Leg press: 180kg	Core stab: -2mmhg	Body fat % 14%	Flex: +16

RE-TEST TARGETS: IN 12 WEEKS

VO$_2$max: 60mlO2/kg/min	OBLA: 17km/hr	Chest press: 115kg	Leg press: 200kg	Core stab: -4mmhg	Body fat % 12%	Flex: +16

PROGRAMME OVERVIEW:

CV day:	Mon	Tue	Wed	Thur	Fri	Sat	Sun
Target:	20–30 mins 6–8RPE		20–30 mins 6–8RPE				
Achieved:	✓		✓				

Swim:	Mon	Tue	Wed	Thur	Fri	Sat	Sun
Target:	Speed	Power	Speed	Aerobic	Speed	Status dependent	
Achieved:	✓	✓	✓	✓	AS		

Weights:	Mon	Tue	Wed	Thur	Fri	Sat	Sun
Target:	UB1	LB1	UB1	LB1		WB	
Achieved:	✓	✓	AS	✓		✓	

Core:	Mon	Tue	Wed	Thur	Fri	Sat	Sun
Target:		CS1	CS1	CS1	CS1		
Achieved:		✓	✓	✗	✓		

Key: ✓ = completed prescribed session   AS = attempted session   X = Did not do session

Client notes:
Took part in Friday's speed session but couldn't keep up as felt tired. Did most of the session but only at about 80% effort. Didn't complete Wed's UB session as didn't feel strong enough. Missed Thursday's core session due to dental appointment. Overall felt cardio intensities were at the right level but would prefer 20 mins cardio rather than 30.

Plan of action:
Agree to target 20 mins cardio to reduce impact on Friday's speed session. Reduce weight (increase RM) for Wed's UB session to allow for recovery from Monday.

Figure 7.3 Weekly programme monitoring form. (For a blank template please visit: www.bloomsbury.com/9781408187234)

of the next testing session – often a useful visual reminder for the client, and very motivating.

Contacting the trainer

As the way in which all sessions and programmes are delivered will differ from client to client it is important that the way in which the client contacts the trainer is agreed at the start of the programme. This information can also be recorded on the session card to act as a reminder for the client should they need to contact the trainer between sessions.

PROGRAMME MONITORING

For the benefit of both the trainer and the client it is important that each individual exercise session is monitored so that the trainer is able to assess progression of health and fitness components in relation to any agreed goals or targets and adapt the programme to suit.

There are many methods used in the health and fitness industry to monitor the progress of exercise programmes. A simple way to do this is to use a recording method such as the weekly programme monitoring form, as shown in figure 7.3 The weekly programme monitoring form should be explained to the client during the initial client review meeting, prior to the induction session. Clients should be asked to complete the form by indicating (using the key) whether they completed, attempted or did not attend the prescribed session and then provide this for the trainer at the follow-up review meetings. They should also be encouraged to make notes relating to their views as it is not always possible for the trainer to be at every session and client feedback is important in relation to exercise adherence and programme success.

PROGRAMME REVIEW AND ADAPTATION

Periodic programme reviews are essential to the outcome of exercise programmes for many reasons:

1. They allow clients to express their personal views and opinions.
2. They provide an opportunity for clients to give feedback in relation to specific exercises in each individual session.
3. They allow discussion to take place between client and trainer in relation to programme issues.
4. They provide information relating to individual session on which to base any required programme adaptations.
5. They are an accurate record of any programme changes that have been made in relation to H&F components.
6. They allow the trainer to make informed programme changes in a timely manner.
7. They provide an opportunity for trainer's to give feedback to clients in relation to programme changes that might have been made.

The frequency of review meetings is something that should be discussed between the trainer and the client but it is advised that weekly meetings take place in order to make any necessary programme changes. Completed weekly programme monitoring forms can be discussed at the review meetings to help agree action plans for forthcoming sessions. This gives the client the opportunity to re-assess their own goals should they feel it necessary.

When reviewing weekly monitoring forms, check that each health and fitness component has fulfilled fitness principles such as frequency, time, intensity, etc., and only make any changes that are necessary. If it is apparent that goals are not being met or where new goals have been identified, then each component of health and fitness should be addressed and adjusted in line with the appropriate principles of fitness (see page 39).

The trainer should make sure that overall long-term goals and medium-term objectives are available at review meetings so that weekly achievements can be compared against them and any changes are made, if necessary. If any changes are made to the programme, this is recorded on the appropriate form, such as the PT session card or weekly profile. Trainers should always keep any information relating to an individual exercise programme as well as recording any changes to the programme that have been made in order to have a record of how any changes to a programme affected the client's goals. This could help inform any decisions that might be made in the future. If no changes to the programme are to be made, trainers are advised to reinforce to clients that the programme is 'on-track', which will increase the chances of them achieving their individual goals that were agreed at the start of the process.

TRAINING METHODS

8

THE NOS LEVEL 3 PERSONAL TRAINER CRITERIA COVERED IN THIS CHAPTER ARE:

- The different training systems and their use in providing variety and ensuring programmes remain effective
- How timings, intensities and sequences can affect outcomes

TRAINING METHODS

Once a client has started a regular exercise programme, one of their main concerns is that they might get bored or the programme starts to feel stale. Trainers should include variety in their clients' programmes in order to maintain motivation and effectiveness.

The range of training methods available to the trainer is vast (and beyond the scope of this book) and the choice of exercises is often based on the preference of the trainer and the availability of resources. For this reason it may be easier for the trainer to think of the current thinking in relation to each fitness components. The components that will be discussed in this chapter are aerobic, anaerobic, muscular strength, muscular power, muscular endurance (including stabilisation) and flexibility.

AEROBIC OR ENDURANCE TRAINING

Aerobic training is so called as it is predominantly the aerobic energy system that is being targeted. The optimal combination of intensity and volume required to produce the greatest aerobic fitness improvements depends on many factors, such as the individual's initial fitness levels, genetics, age, weight, etc. Training intensities for endurance athletes typically range from 60–100% of VO_2max. Many elite athletes exercise at an intensity sufficiently high enough to recruit fast twitch type II fibres (particularly for shorter endurance events) whereas many recreational individuals remain at levels that recruit mainly slow twitch type I fibres. In order to cater for the wide variety of endurance events/sports, endurance training intensities can be categorised into easy recovery efforts, long and steady state,

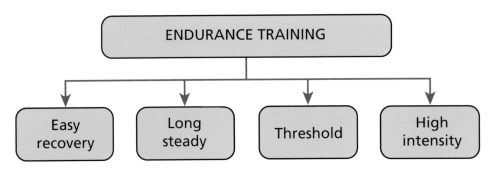

Figure 8.1 Typical endurance training zones

threshold training and high-intensity training (HIT) as can be seen in figure 8.1

- *Easy recovery* – easy recovery sessions are typically used to recover both physiologically and psychologically from any previous hard training sessions. The mode of exercise does not have to be the same as that used in the previous endurance session. For example, runners often swim or cycle in recovery sessions.
- *Long and steady* – otherwise known as Long Slow Distance (LSD) training, sessions typically last between 1–2 hours at intensities of approximately 60–70% VO_2max. As all individuals respond differently it is important to keep the intensity below anaerobic threshold

level (the transition between aerobic and anaerobic levels).

- *Threshold training* – this is essentially training just below and just above anaerobic threshold. Threshold training in addition to long and steady exercise has been demonstrated to improve running economy (efficiency of movement) which is useful in almost every sport.
- *High Intensity Training (HIT)* – these are essentially interval training sessions that mimic the work-to-rest ratios that are typical of the specific sport or event of the client. The work-to-rest ratio is dependent on many factors however; general guidelines are shown in table 8.1.

Table 8.1 Typical work-to-rest ratios for HIT zones

Intensity (HIT zone)	Work to rest ratio	Work duration	Rest duration
95–100%	1:3	Up to 10 seconds	15–30 seconds
85–90%	1:2	10–45 seconds	0.5–1.5 mins
75–85%	1:1	45 secs–2 mins	1.5–2 mins

Table 8.2   Physiological adaptations to endurance-type training

Zone	Main adaptations
Long steady	**Central adaptations:** Increases in blood volume, left ventricle size and stroke volume resulting in increased cardiac output and oxygen delivery to the muscles. **Peripheral adaptations:** Increased muscle capillary density, number and size of mitochondria and aerobic enzymes. Slow twitch type I fibres increase in size. Fast twitch type IIb fibres can be converted to more fatigue resistance fast twitch type IIa fibres. The net result is greater fat breakdown and reduced reliance on limited muscle glycogen stores.
Threshold	A decrease in lactate production and an increase in lactate removal. Greater re-synthesis of ATP from aerobic sources resulting in reduced reliance on anaerobic glycolysis.
HIT	Only some studies have found VO_2max improvements, explained as a result of decreased lactate production at a fixed workload.

Individuals new to interval training should have a good cardio base and begin with the maximum recommended rest period specific to the intensity of the exercise performed. Gradually reduce the rest period as they become accustomed to the training. Medium and long work-to-rest ratio training sessions have been shown to be physiologically more demanding (and show a greater utilisation of carbohydrates) than short work-to-rest ratio sessions.

Physiological adaptations to aerobic training

There are many physiological adaptations that occur as a result of endurance-type training. Table 8.2 summarises the main adaptations in relation to the endurance training zones.

ANAEROBIC TRAINING

Exercising at intensity levels approaching 100% VO_2max or above is referred to as anaerobic training as the anaerobic energy systems are predominantly used. For programming purposes anaerobic training is sometimes divided into short-term or long-term depending on the anaerobic energy systems targeted (ATP-PC and anaerobic glycolysis – see chapter 8). Short-term anaerobic endurance training as it is better known is designed to increase the ability to perform maximal work for a short period of time and long-term anaerobic endurance training is designed to improve the ability to maintain exercise at a high intensity.

Short-term anaerobic endurance training

One of the main goals of short-term anaerobic training is to develop the capacity of the ATP-PC

Table 8.3	Typical training for short-term anaerobic endurance			
	Repetitions		**Distance/Time**	**Recovery**
Running	10		100 metres	3–5 mins
Cycling	10–12 (maximal)		10 seconds	Full recovery
Typical adaptations	• Increase in ATP, creatine and PC stores. • Increase in concentration and activity of enzymes involved in the phosphagen system (creatine kinase and myokinase).			

system. Typically, short duration repetitions of less than 15 seconds should be performed in training sessions to target this energy system. If recovery between repetitions is short enough, the anaerobic glycolysis system will also be targeted. For example, a 1:10 work-to-rest ratio (this simply means that the rest period should be 10 times longer than the work period) between repetitions is often used with a 3–5 minutes or full recovery between sets.

It has been shown that low intensity exercise during recovery periods can help to increase blood flow and aid recovery. Typical details (and adaptations) for running and cycling short-term anaerobic endurance training can be seen in table 8.3

Long-term anaerobic endurance training

The main goal of long-term anaerobic endurance training is to develop the anaerobic glycolysis system (and slow down the lactic acid produced when using this energy system). Repetitions of between 30–180 seconds duration are typically performed with work-to-rest ratios of 1:4 and 1:5 with a long or full recovery (see table 8.4). Alternatively shorter bouts of exercise (20–120 seconds) with shorter rest periods and 1:1 work-to-rest ratios (termed lactate tolerance training)

can be used. If the client is training for a particular sport or event, the trainer should try to match the work-to-rest ratio to his or her specific demands. An example of typical training details (and adaptations) for running and cycling long-term anaerobic endurance training can be seen in table 8.4.

Physiological adaptations to anaerobic training

Adaptations to anaerobic training mainly occur in the muscle groups recruited as a result of the exercises performed during the training, however, the better the aerobic system, the better the recovery from high-intensity exercise. Main adaptations can be seen in tables 8.3 and 8.4.

RESISTANCE TRAINING

There are many methods of resistance training but no one method is ideal for the entire population, therefore, the method should be tailored to suit the goals of the individual. It may be necessary to try a certain resistance training method for a period of time in order to evaluate the effectiveness in relation to the goals of the individual. An example of just some of the more commonly used resistance training methods can be seen in table 8.5.

Table 8.4 Typical training for long-term anaerobic endurance

	Repetitions		Distance/Time	Recovery
Running	10–12		100 metres	30–60 seconds
Running	8		400 metres	3 minutes
Cycling	10–12		30 seconds	4–5 minutes
Typical adaptations	• Increase in concentration and activity of enzymes involved in the anaerobic glycolysis system (phosphofructokinase). • Increased capacity to buffer acid production within the muscle and the blood.			

Table 8.5 Commonly used training methods

Training method	Description
Single sets	Performing one set on each exercise.
Multiple sets	Performing more than one set on each exercise.
Circuit sets	A series of resistance exercises with a rest period between each exercise.
Super sets	Performing several exercises for the same body part or pairing exercises for agonist and antagonist.
Pyramids	Increasing the resistance and decreasing the repetitions over several sets.
Delorme-Watkins	This system involves increasing the intensity based on 10RM. For example, if a client has a 10RM of 40kg for the shoulder press, they would perform: Set 1 – 10 reps of 50% of 10RM = 20kg Set 2 – 10 reps of 75% of 10RM = 30kg Set 3 – 10 reps of 100% of 10RM = 40kg
7s, 14s and 21s	Sets that include multiples of 7.
Drop sets	Continuous lowering of the resistance with fatigue at each set.
Complex training	Combination of resistance training and plyometrics.

Kinetic chain

Resistance exercises are sometimes divided into two broad categories: Open Kinetic Chain (OKCE) and Closed Kinetic Chain exercises (CKCE).

OKCE can be described as exercises in which the load or resistance is moving in relation to the body (for example, knee-extensions or lat pull-downs using resistance machines). CKCE can be described as exercises in which the body is moving in relation to the load (for example the front and back squat, lunge and pull-up). There is much debate in this area but it is generally accepted that CKCE exercises are better for sporting movements or everyday lifestyle activities as they typically involve the body moving against gravity. In terms of exercise selection, trainers should try and match exercises to the specific demands of the clients' sport or event and in particular to the category of OKCE or CKCE.

Another area that the trainer should consider in terms of resistance exercises is that of intensity and volume.

Intensity and volume selection

Training intensity (otherwise known as the 'load') is often expressed as the repetition maximum or RM (maximum weight lifted for a specific number of repetitions, e.g. 3RM is the maximum weight that can be lifted for 3 repetitions). Intensity can also be expressed as a percentage of 1RM (e.g. 80% of 1RM). Training volume is the term used to describe the total work performed per session and is typically calculated as sets x repetitions x load. For example, for an individual who performs 3 sets of 10 repetitions of 80kg, the volume can be calculated as 3 x 10 x 80 = 2400kg. Training volume is considered to be one of the major factors effecting strength or muscle mass gains. The intensity and volume of the load should depend

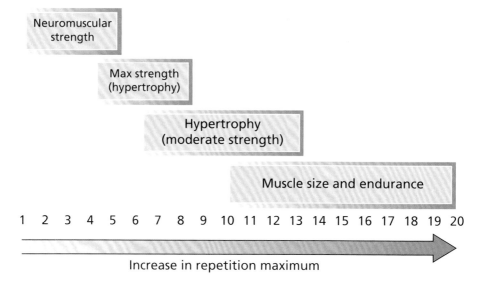

Figure 8.2 Strength endurance continuum related to RM

Table 8.6	Strength training recommendations for novice intermediate and advanced		
	Novice	**Intermediate**	**Advanced**
Intensity (% of max)	50–60	60–80	80–100
Sets	1–2	2–3	2–5
Reps	10–15	8–12	1–8
Frequency (Sessions per week)	1–2	2–3	3–5
Rest (minutes)	1.5	2	3

on the goal in terms of strength, power or endurance. The strength-endurance continuum shows how the number of repetitions can be related to goal outcomes (figure 8.2).

Maximum strength gains typically occur following training programmes that incorporate loads between 1 and 10RM, although not all training can be at this intensity, due to the risk of overtraining and injury. Training for hypertrophy or power is normally done in the range between 8 and 15RM and endurance between 12 and 20RM (although note the overlap due to many varying factors). During inductions the trainer should determine the weight that corresponds to the RM chosen for the client for each exercise.

Trainers should also have a good understanding of the literature pertaining to muscular strength, muscular power and muscular endurance.

Muscular strength

Even though there is still no consensus opinion regarding a single definition of the term 'strength', it is often linked to the ability to lift heavy weights by the recruitment of fast twitch type II fibres.

The optimal resistance training programme (with respect to intensity, volume, rest, etc.) does not exist due to varying responses of different individuals. Strength training often uses progressively increasing resistances and often results in hypertrophy even though it is possible to gain strength without concomitant gains in muscle size. Exercises can be performed using different methods of muscular contraction such as isometric (equal length), concentric (toward the middle), eccentric (away from the middle) and a combination of all. All methods have been shown to elicit strength gains, therefore, trainers should try to match exercises to specific goals, however, table 8.6 shows a general recommendation in relation to strength training for novice, intermediate and advanced individuals.

Muscular power

In the context of resistance training, muscular power can be thought of as a combination of strength and speed. It is generally agreed that muscular strength should be developed before training for muscular power. Typically, light to moderate loads lifted at speed are used extensively in training programmes to develop muscular power for specific sports or athletic events. However, this has been challenged by Bruce-Low and Smith (2006), who state that evidence does not support the view that such exercises are more effective than traditional, slow and heavy weight training in enhancing muscle power and athletic performance. If light to moderate training loads are used to develop muscular power, trainers should make sure that strength training should be reduced during these periods in order to avoid any detrimental effects (power training should come before strength training if done in the same session). Trainers should also note that clients should have a good strength base before undertaking any power training. Although muscular power training is dependent on the sport or event being trained for, resistance training can be carried out using general recommendations as shown in table 8.7.

Another common training method that is often used (and also challenged by Bruce-Low and Smith) for the development of muscular power is that of 'plyometric' training.

PLYOMETRIC TRAINING

One of the methods of training that is often used by sports people or athletes to develop muscular power is called 'plyometric' training. Derived from Greek meaning 'changing length', plyometric can be defined as 'rapid eccentric loading (the muscle stretching quickly) followed by a brief isometric phase (no muscle shortening or lengthening) and explosive rebound (the muscle shortening quickly) using stored elastic energy and powerful concentric contractions'. This can be further explained by separating a plyometric movement into phases as in table 8.8.

During the eccentric or loading phase the muscle fibres are stretched rapidly which causes a response known as the 'stretch reflex' (see page 123) which then initiates a contraction (or development of tension) in the fibres of the same muscle. Plyometric exercises must be performed rapidly as the

Table 8.7	General power training recommendations		
	Set I	Set 2	Set 3
Intensity (% of IRM)	70	60	50
Reps	4–6	6–8	8–10
Rest (minutes)	2–2.5	3	3.5

Table 8.8	Plyometric phases
Phase	**Description**
Eccentric (loading)	This is where the prime mover lengthens.
Amortisation	This is the brief period when the prime mover has stretched to full length and before any contraction.
Concentric (unloading)	This is the shortening of the prime mover.

stretch reflex response takes only 0.2 seconds to occur. The time between the two phases, known as the 'amortisation' phase allows for the build up of elastic energy. The elastic property of connective tissue (muscle and tendon) is also thought to contribute to power development. Stretching of the connective tissue during eccentric muscle contraction produces a store of potential energy, and when this energy is released during the concentric phase of the muscular contraction, it helps to augment the power of that contraction.

De-sensitisation of the Golgi Tendon Organ is thought to allow a greater force development but this is not discussed here. When done quickly as explained before, this plyometric movement is known as the stretch shortening cycle (SCC). It has been demonstrated that plyometric training programmes have improved performance in areas such as vertical jump, anaerobic peak power, and maximum squat as a result of physiological changes. The trainer must be aware, however, that precautions must be taken with this type of high-intensity training especially with children and those with no history of previous resistance training.

Plyometric guidelines
Guidelines for plyometric training are normally recommended to minimise the risk of musculoskeletal injury. Before including this type of training in a client programme the trainer should consider the following areas.

Strength base
Clients should have a good strength base due to the intense nature of the plyometric exercises. Strength ratios of 1.5 to 2.5 times body weight for 1RM squats (lower body plyometrics) and 1.0 to 1.5 times body weight for bench press (upper body plyometrics) are recommended. Other recommendations include the ability to perform 5 consecutive clap push-ups. If a client does not possess the strength capability for either lower or upper body strength recommendations, then it is suggested that plyometric exercises should be delayed until they do. For beginners to plyometrics, it is important to focus on correct technique prior to any loaded or intense exercises. It is also recommended to start with soft ground outdoors before progression to harder surfaces.

Age
Clients should be at least 16 years to undergo plyometric exercises. However, the American College of Sports Medicine, while not specifying any age requirement, advises that to minimise the likelihood of injury, participants must be closely supervised, learn the correct technique, and training intensity and volume must not exceed the abilities of the participants. Trainers should consider the training history of each client, especially those under the age of 16 years, and make sure that progression for any plyometric exercise programme is slow.

Jump height
Plyometric training often includes the use of box jumps or reactive jumps, whereby the optimal height commonly suggested is between 75 and 110cms (research often shows that plyometric training jumps of over 110cms do not elicit the Stretch Shortening Cycle) .

Rest periods
Plyometric exercises can cause fatigue not only of energy stores but also of the Central Nervous

System (CNS). Work to rest ratios of 1:5 are often quoted as being sufficient for recovery.

Volume

A common way to measure the total amount of work performed during a training session is to count the foot contacts. A general recommendation is that no more than 100 foot contacts per session are exceeded.

Lower-body plyometric exercises

Exercises 8.1 to 8.5 show a selection of lower-body plyometric exercises which are ordered in relation to progression of intensity.

Exercise 8.1 Tuck jump

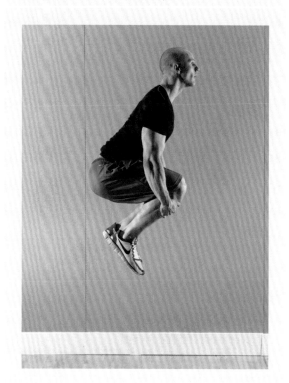

A tuck jump requires the individual landing in the same spot from where they jumped and then taking off again as quickly as possible. Progression can involve the use of weights carried by the jumper.

- Adopt a standing position.
- Perform a small countermovement.
- Jump up, bringing the knees to the chest.
- Land on the balls of the feet and spring up immediately.
- Keep the floor contact time as short as possible.

Exercise 8.2 Bunny hops

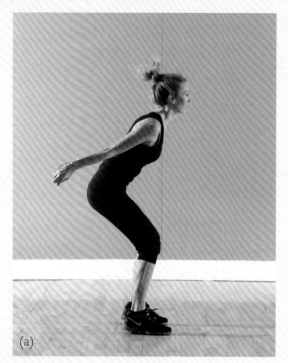 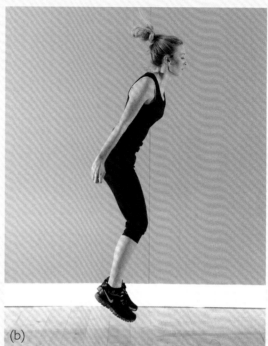

(a)   (b)

Bunny hops require a maximum effort with each repetition as they are done one after another usually for distances of 10–30 metres. Hurdles can be used to help with spacing and height.

- With both feet together, jump forward and land (on balls of the feet) and immediately take off again and repeat.
- Swinging the arms can help to increase the length of the jump.
- Keep the floor contact time as short as possible.

Exercise 8.3 Bounding

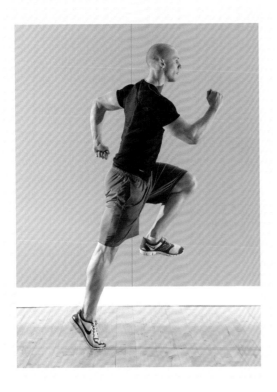

Exercise 8.4 Single-leg hops

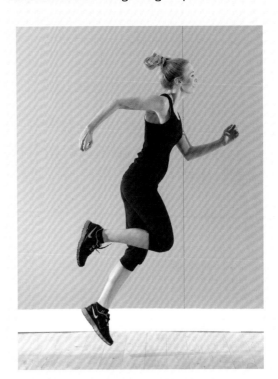

Bounding resembles an exaggerated running stride, which is commonly used in training to improve stride length or stride frequency. Bounds are typically performed for distances greater than 30 metres.

- Progress from a slow jog to an extended running style.
- Make each stride as long as possible and immediately take off again.
- Keep the floor contact time as short as possible.

Single-leg hops require a maximal effort with each repetition as they are done one after another on the same foot usually for distances of 10–30 metres. Hurdles can be used to help with spacing and height.

- Push off with one leg and land on the same ball of the foot of the same leg. Immediately take off again and repeat.
- Swinging the opposite leg can help to increase the length of the jump.
- Floor contact time as short as possible.
- For progression, try to pull the heel toward the buttocks during the jump.

Exercise 8.5 Depth jumps

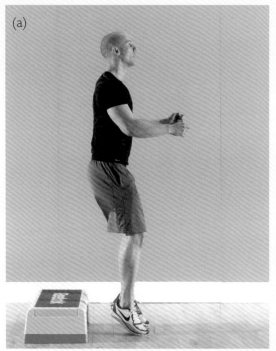
(a)

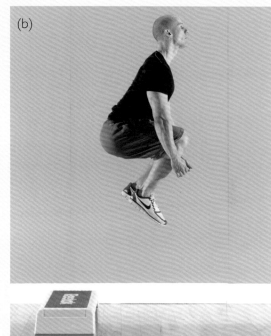
(b)

Depth jumps are performed by stepping off a box and attempting to jump up as high as possible.

- Stand on the box with the toes close to the front edge.
- Step from the box and land on balls of the feet.
- Keep the contact time on the ground short by springing up in the air as soon as possible.

Upper-body plyometric exercises

Exercises 8.6 to 8.8 show a selection of upper-body plyometric exercises which are ordered in relation to progression of intensity.

Exercise 8.6 Chest pass

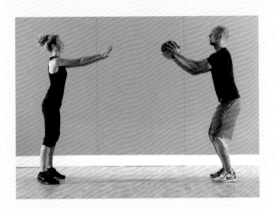

Medicine or weighted balls are needed for this exercise where the number of repetitions depends on how long it takes for the shoulders to become fatigued. Try leaning back to angle the body at 45 degrees to vary the exercise.

- Face a partner with feet shoulder-width apart and knees slightly bent.
- Begin by holding the medicine ball with both hands at chest level, elbows pointing out.
- Push the medicine ball away from the chest and extend the arms.
- With arms extended, catch the ball and bring it towards the chest before repeating the throw again.
- Keep the catch and throw time as short as possible.

Exercise 8.7 Power drop

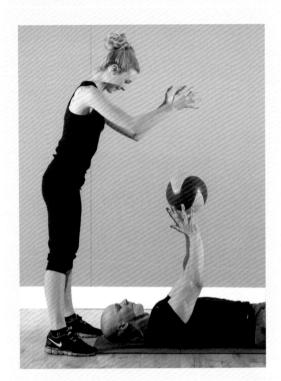

This exercise isolates the pectoral muscles, as opposed to the chest press which incorporates many stabilising muscles.

- Lie supine on the ground with the arms outstretched.
- As the partner drops the medicine ball, catch the ball with elbows bent.
- Allow the ball to come towards your chest.
- Extend the arms to propel the ball back to the partner on the box.
- Keep the catch time to the shortest time possible.

Exercise 8.8 Rotation throw

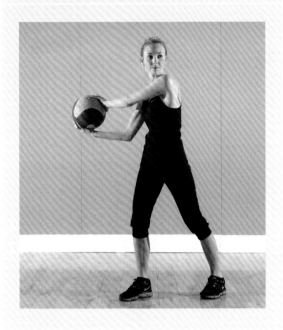

Used to develop power in throwing movements, medicine balls should be used with the weight appropriate to the client. Good core stabilisation is required for this exercise.

- Stand with feet shoulder-width apart and upright posture.
- Bend the catching arm about 90 degrees with elbow into the side.
- Externally rotate the catching arm ready to catch the ball but keep the trunk facing forward.
- A partner throws a small medicine ball (1–2kg) to the catching hand.
- On catching the ball take it across the body by internally rotating the catching arm then immediately throw the ball back by externally rotating the catching arm.
- Repeat for the opposite arm.

Exercise 8.9 Clap push-up

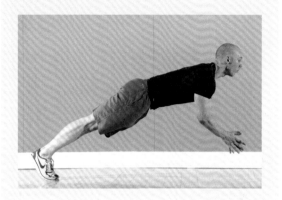

This is a progression from the chest press or power drop as there is a great deal of strength required for this exercise.

- Adopt a push-up position with the hands approximately shoulder-width apart.
- Push off from the ground, clap the hands, then land with both hands back to the starting position.
- Keep the floor contact time as short as possible.

Exercise 8.10 Incline push-up depth jump

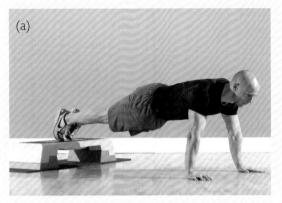 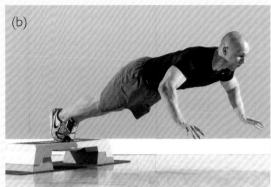

This exercise requires good upper-body strength and good core stabilisation. Do not perform with any type of wrist injury or weakness.

- Place two mats about shoulder-width apart.
- Use a box to raise the feet slightly above shoulder height.
- Adopt a push-up position with the feet on the box and hands between the mats.
- Push off from the ground and land with one hand on each mat then as quickly as possible push off the mats with both hands back to the starting position.
- Keep the floor contact time as short as possible.

MUSCULAR ENDURANCE

The term muscular endurance is sometimes referred to as 'power endurance' and is linked to the recruitment of slow twitch type I fibres. As endurance can be very diverse in relation to both number of repetitions and outcomes, trainers and coaches are recommended to replicate the demands of the sport in training programmes. Muscular endurance can be thought of in two ways: firstly, to perform repeated contractions against resistance over a period of time, and, secondly, to create muscular tension over a long period of time (stabilisation). Resistance training for muscular endurance is often associated with a high number of repetitions using a comparatively low weight or resistance. As with all types of resistance training, there are many methods employed for targeting muscular endurance depending on the event and the individual. Table 8.9 shows general recommendations for muscular endurance resistance training.

Another method of training that is also associated with muscular endurance is that of stabilisation.

Stabilisation

Muscles that perform predominantly a stabilisation role in a given situation are often referred to as 'stabilisers' (also known as tonic muscles).

Due to the demands of endurance-type tasks, stabilisers are predominantly made up of type I slow-twitch fibres. Muscles that are mainly responsible for large movements of the body are commonly known as 'mobilisers' (also known as phasic muscles). These muscles are usually required to provide a short-term role and are therefore predominantly made up of fast-twitch fibres and are closer to the surface than stabiliser muscles. It should be noted that all muscles can provide a certain degree of joint stabilisation but only certain muscles can provide locomotion.

Sometimes stabilising and mobilising muscles are trained in the opposite role from that for which they were designed. For example, the rectus abdominis is predominantly a fast-twitch muscle close to the surface of the body and is normally active in strength or explosive tasks, such as running and jumping where the legs come towards the torso (spinal flexion). However, it is common for exercise programmes to include sit-up type exercises that are performed repetitively in an endurance-type capacity. The rectus abdominis (and hip flexors) is mainly responsible for this sit-up action, which effectively results in a predominantly fast-twitch muscle being trained as a slow-twitch muscle, which is thought can lead to a weakness of the stabiliser muscles

Table 8.9	General muscular endurance training recommendations		
	Short term	**Medium term**	**Long term**
Reps	12–25	25–50	50–100
Sets	3	2–3	1–2
Rest	30–60 secs	1–1.5 mins	1.5–2 mins
Method	Light weights	Bands, med balls, etc.	Body weight

Table 8.10 Muscles associated with stabilisation of the core, hip and shoulder

Area of stabilisation	Main stabiliser muscles
Core or trunk area	Stabiliser muscles with little mobilisation ability: • Transversus abdominis • Multifidus • Pelvic floor • Diaphragm • Internal obliques • Quadratus lumborum Muscles with a greater mobilisation ability: • Rectus abdominis • External oblique • Erector spinae
Hip	Stabiliser muscles with little mobilisation ability: • Gluteus medius and minimus • Piriformis • Gemellus (inferior and superior) • Obturator (internus and externus) • Quadratus femorus Muscles with a greater mobilisation ability: • Gluteus maximus • Iliopsoas • Tensor fasciae latae • Hamstrings • Adductors • Rectus femoris
Shoulder	Provides stabilisation mainly of the scapula: • Rhomboid • Trapezius • Serratus anterior • Subscapualaris Provides stabilisation mainly of the humeral head: • Infraspinatus • Teres minor/major • Supraspinatous

leading to potential back pain or injury (Richardson *et al*, 2003).

Muscles involved in stabilisation

Muscles in the body can also be classified as deep (also known as *local*) or, in relation to core stabilisation, as the *inner unit*. Muscles that are superficial are commonly known as *global muscles* or the *outer unit*. Although some muscles can have a dual role depending on the circumstances, table 8.10 lists the main muscles generally associated with stabilisation of the core, hip and shoulder.

As core stability is an important aspect of personal training, trainers should have a good understanding of the location of the muscles of the core in relation to stabilising and mobilising.

Transversus abdominis

This muscle forms a belt or corset around the trunk region and lies deep below the rectus abdominis muscle, which is associated with the 'six-pack'. Imagine a belt running underneath the navel, right around the body. This is the transversus abdominis muscle (see figure 8.3).

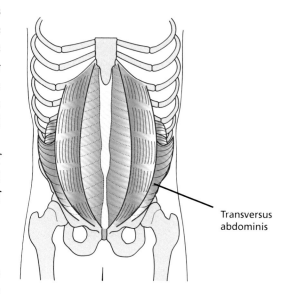

Figure 8.3 Transversus abdominis

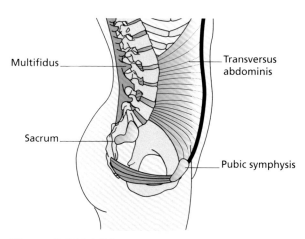

Figure 8.4 Multifidus

Multifidus

This is a series of many small muscles that attach between each vertebra of the spine (see figure 8.4). These muscles act as a kind of lashing for the bones in the spine to prevent any excessive movement.

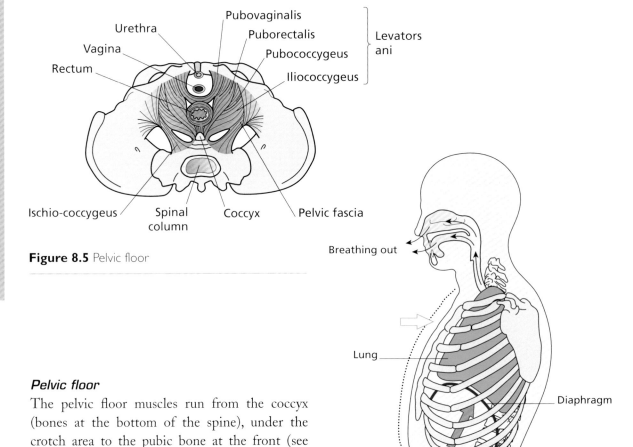

Figure 8.5 Pelvic floor

Breathing out

Lung

Diaphragm

Figure 8.6 Diaphragm

Pelvic floor

The pelvic floor muscles run from the coccyx (bones at the bottom of the spine), under the crotch area to the pubic bone at the front (see figure 8.5).

Diaphragm

This is a dome-shaped muscle that covers the region under the ribcage (see figure 8.6). As well as performing core stabilisation tasks, the diaphragm is responsible for helping in breathing movements.

Internal obliques

These attach from the lower ribs and insert into the pubic bone, and lie at an angle just above and below the navel (see figure 8.7). They are quite deep and cannot be seen superficially.

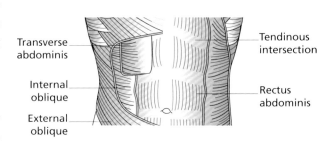

Figure 8.7 Internal obliques

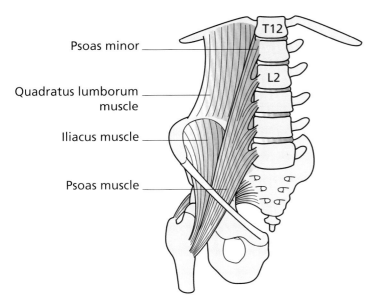

Figure 8.8 Quadratus lumborum

Psoas minor

Quadratus lumborum muscle

Iliacus muscle

Psoas muscle

T12

L2

Quadratus lumborum

This muscle runs from the iliac crest to the transverse processes of the upper 4 lumbar vertebrae and also attaches to the twelfth rib (see figure 8.8). It is quite a deep muscle that is associated with side bends (i.e. bringing the ribs closer to the pelvis).

Rectus abdominis

This muscle runs the length of the abdomen from the ribs down to the pubic bone and is held in place by fascia running horizontally across the muscle, which gives it the appearance of having sections (see figure 8.9).

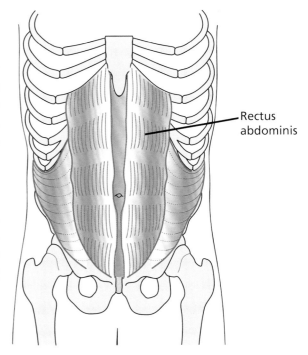

Rectus abdominis

Figure 8.9 Rectus abdominis

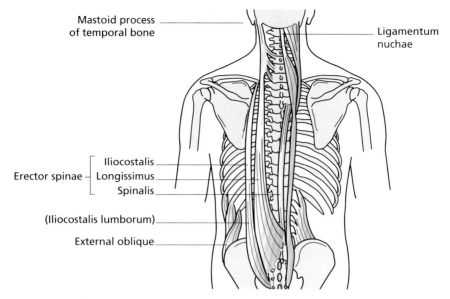

Figure 8.10 Erector spinae

Erector spinae

This is a group of individual muscles that run either side of the spine from the sacrum and iliac crest to the base of the skull (see figure 8.10).

External obliques

This superficial muscle lies almost at a vertical angle and runs from the surface of the lower 8 ribs down to the iliac crest (see figure 8.11).

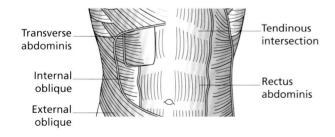

Figure 8.11 External obliques

Stabilisation exercises

Most trainers will be familiar with mobiliser-type exercises but may be less familiar with stabiliser-type exercises. There are no definitive guidelines in relation to stabilisation exercises using body weight as resistance, therefore, the trainer should use common sense and treat each client individually. As a general guide, stabilisation exercises are usually carried out between 15 and 30 seconds with the number of repetitions dependent on the individual in relation to loss of form or fatigue. Exercises 8.11 to 8.20 are examples of some of the common exercises (using either the floor or a stability ball) for targeting muscles used for core stabilisation.

Exercise 8.11 Kneeling abdominal hollow

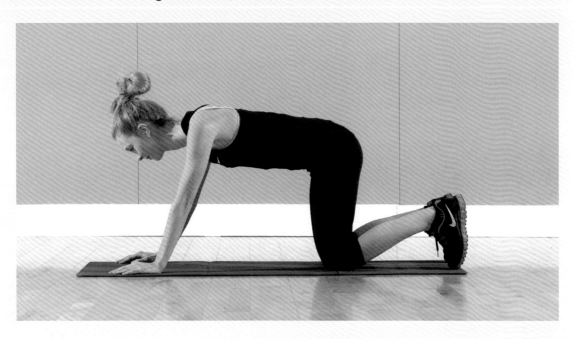

Starting position
- Kneel on the floor with your shoulders directly above your hands and your hips directly above your knees.
- Keep your head facing down towards the floor to prevent undue stress on the cervical spine.
- Keep your knees shoulder-width apart. Check that your spine is in the neutral position.

Action
- Consciously contract your transversus abdominis.
- Breathe gently in and out, maintaining the contraction.
- Breathe out and, before breathing in again, try to hollow your lower abdominals (imagine pulling your navel towards your spine).
- Continuing to breathe normally, hold this position for a few seconds or until you are unable to hold it any more.
- Repeat, trying to maintain normal breathing throughout.
- Concentrate on maintaining the starting position during the course of the exercise.

Progressions
- Try to perform the action without contracting the rectus abdominis.
- Once you are comfortable with performing abdominal hollowing on all fours, try to perform the action in a standing position.
- Try to contract the transversus abdominis without drawing in the lower abdominals. This is known as *abdominal bracing*.

113

Exercise 8.12 Supine foot slide

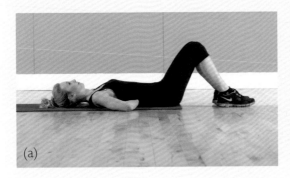
(a)

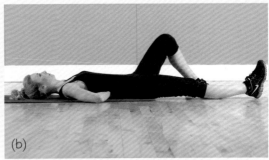
(b)

Starting position

- Lie on your back with your feet flat on the floor and your knees bent as much as is comfortably possible.
- Place one arm down by your side and the other under the lumbar spine to check the pressure on your hand throughout the exercise.
- Keep your knees shoulder-width apart. Check that your spine is in the neutral position.

Action

- Consciously contract your transversus abdominis.
- Breathe gently in and out.
- Slowly slide one foot outwards along the floor until your leg is fully extended.
- Return to the start position, trying to maintain normal breathing throughout.
- Concentrate on keeping your spine in the neutral position during the exercise so that the pressure on your hand does not change.

Progressions

- Once you are comfortable with the above action, try increasing the speed of the movement slightly.
- Once you can perform the above exercise without a change in pressure on the hand under the lumbar spine, try sliding both legs out and back at the same time.

Exercise 8.13 Pelvic tilt.

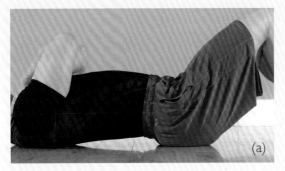
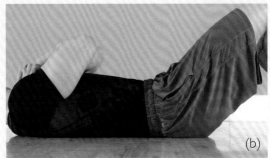

(a)   (b)

Starting position
- Lie on your back with your feet flat on the floor and your knees bent as much as is comfortably possible.
- Place your arms by your sides or across your abdomen.
- Keep your knees shoulder-width apart. Check that your spine is in the neutral position.

Action
- Consciously contract your transversus abdominis.
- Breathe in and out gently.
- Tilt your pelvis backward so that your lower back is flat on the floor (see 8.13 (b)).
- Return to the starting position, trying to maintain normal breathing throughout.

Progressions
- Try performing the exercise while lifting one foot slightly off the floor.
- As well as tilting the pelvis backward, try to tilt it forward so that your lumbar spine is more arched than normal.

Exercise 8.14 Side bridge

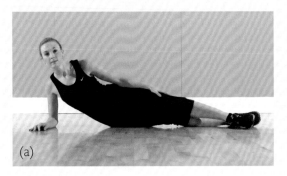

(a)

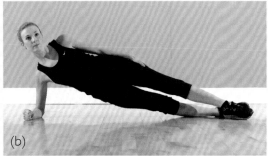

(b)

Starting position

- Lie on your side with your feet slightly apart to create a stable base.
- Bend the arm nearest the floor at the elbow and rest it on the floor. This will provide support when you lift your upper body off the floor.
- Put the opposite arm down by your side. Check that your spine is in the neutral position.
- Keep your upper hip in line with your lower hip (see 8.14 (a)).

Action

- Consciously contract your transversus abdominis.
- Breathe gently in and out.
- Raise your lower hip off the floor so that your body forms a straight line (see 8.14 (b)).
- Hold this position until you start to feel muscle fatigue.
- Try to maintain normal breathing throughout.
- Concentrate on keeping your spine in the neutral position during the exercise.

Progression

- Once you are comfortable with the above exercise, start with the hip in the raised position. Try to lower the hip nearest the floor towards the floor, then raise it to the start position again. Repeat.

Exercise 8.15 Prone plank

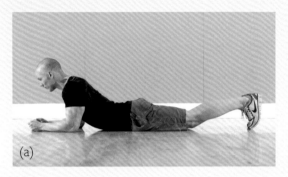
(a)

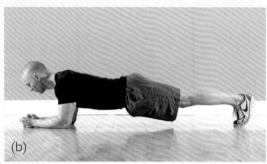
(b)

Starting position
- Lie on your front with your feet slightly apart to create a stable base.
- Place your forearms on the floor with your hands approximately at face level. This will provide support when you lift your body off the floor (see 8.15 (a)).

Action
- Consciously contract your transversus abdominis.
- Breathe gently in and out.
- Raise your body off the floor so that your body forms a straight line (see 8.15 (b)).
- Hold this position until you start to feel muscle fatigue.
- Try to maintain normal breathing throughout.
- Concentrate on keeping your spine in the neutral position during the exercise.

Progression
- Once you are comfortable with the above exercise, try a plank position with straight arms.

Exercise 8.16 Supine plank

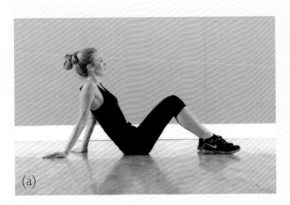

(a)

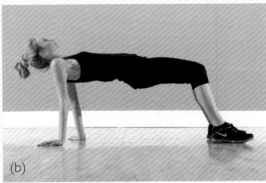

(b)

Starting position

- Lie on your back with your feet slightly apart to create a stable base.
- Bend your knees to approximately 90 degrees and keep your feet flat on the floor and your arms by your side. This will provide support when you lift your body off the floor (8.16 (a)).

Action

- Consciously contract your transversus abdominis.
- Breathe gently in and out.
- Raise your body off the floor so that your body forms a straight line (see 8.16 (b)).
- Hold this position until you start to feel muscle fatigue.
- Try to maintain normal breathing throughout.
- Concentrate on keeping your spine in the neutral position during the exercise.

Progression

- Once you are comfortable with the above exercise, try keeping the plank position but raise one leg straight out in front. You could also try both positions with the arms across the chest.

Exercise 8.17 Shoulder bridge

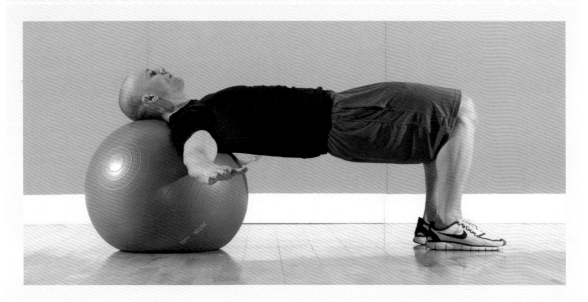

Starting position

- Sit upright on the ball.
- Walk your feet forward and lean back at the same time until the ball is under your shoulder blades.
- Lie face up with the ball under your shoulder blades.
- Rest your head back onto the ball.
- Keep your feet shoulder-width apart and your arms outstretched with the palms facing down.
- Check that your spine is in the neutral position.
- Keep a straight horizontal line through your shoulder, knee and hip joints.

Action

- Consciously contract your transversus abdominis.
- With your feet shoulder-width apart and your arms outstretched, gently roll a few inches to one side at the shoulders, then return to the start point.
- Repeat, but roll to the opposite side.
- Repeat this five times to each side.
- Maintain normal breathing throughout.
- Concentrate on maintaining the starting position during the exercise.

Safety point

Roll only as far as you feel in control of the movement. Use your hands to prevent yourself rolling if you go too far.

Exercise 8.18 Straight leg bridge

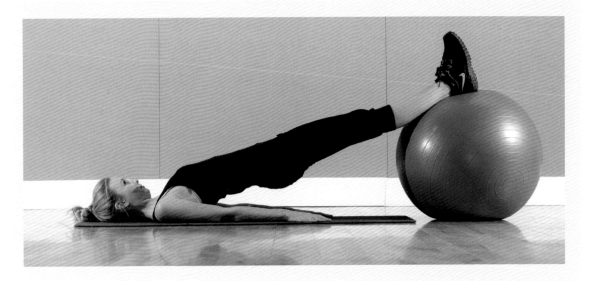

Starting position

- Lie face up on the floor.
- Place the ball under your feet just below your heels.
- Keep your feet shoulder-width apart and your arms outstretched.
- Raise your bottom off the floor until your spine is in the neutral position.
- There should be a straight line through the knee and hip joint.
- Only your shoulder blades, head and arms should be resting on the floor.

Action

- Consciously contract your transversus abdominis.
- With your feet shoulder-width apart and your arms outstretched, use your feet to roll the ball gently a few inches to one side, then return to the starting point.
- Repeat, but roll to the opposite side.
- Repeat five times to each side.
- Maintain normal breathing throughout.
- Concentrate on maintaining the starting position during the exercise.

Safety point

Roll only as far as you feel in control of the movement. If you lose control, adopt the starting position and repeat from the point at which you lost control.

Exercise 8.19 Front bridge

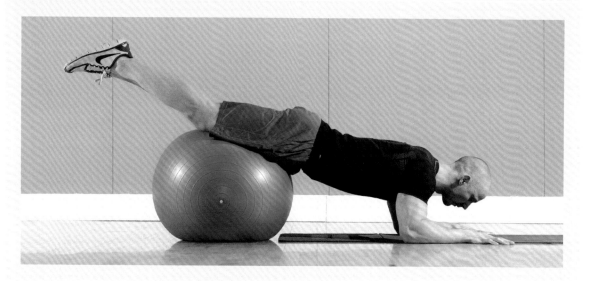

Starting position
- Kneel on the floor in front of the ball.
- Lean forward over the ball so that your chest rests on the ball.
- Roll over the top of the ball so that your forearms rest on the floor in front of the ball and your pelvis rests directly on top of the ball.
- Check that your spine is in the neutral position.
- Keep your neck in neutral by looking down at the floor.
- Maintain a straight line through your knee, hip and shoulder joints.

Action
- Consciously contract your transversus abdominis.
- With your feet together and your forearms on the floor, gently roll the ball a few inches to one side and then return to the start point.
- Repeat, but roll to the opposite side.
- Repeat five times to each side.
- Maintain normal breathing throughout.
- Concentrate on maintaining the starting position during the exercise.

Safety point
Roll only as far as you feel in control of the movement. Put one foot on the floor if you feel you are about to lose control.

Exercise 8.20 Ab-burner

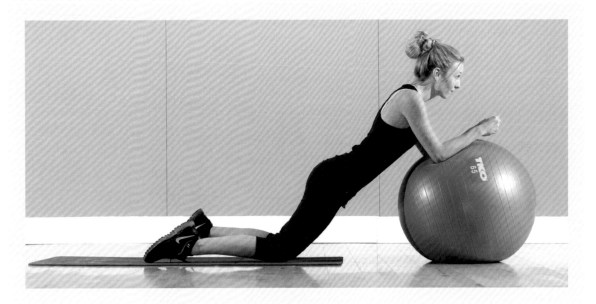

Starting position
- Kneel on the floor about 3 feet in front of the ball.
- Lean forward over the ball so that your forearms rest on the ball.
- Keep your knees shoulder-width apart.
- Check that your spine is in the neutral position.
- Keep your neck in neutral by looking at the floor in front of the ball.

Action
- Consciously contract your transversus abdominis.
- With your knees shoulder-width apart and your forearms on the ball, gently roll the ball a few inches to one side and then return to the start point.
- Repeat, but roll to the opposite side.
- Repeat five times to each side.
- Maintain normal breathing throughout.
- Concentrate on maintaining the starting position during the exercise.

Safety point
Roll only as far as you feel in control of the movement. Use your hands to prevent yourself rolling if you go too far.

FLEXIBILITY

The term 'flexibility' is 'the available range of motion around a specific joint', and the term 'stretching' is often described as 'the method or technique used to influence the joint range of motion either acutely or on a permanent basis'. Maintaining good flexibility leads to many benefits, such as a reduction in injury risk and an ability to perform daily functions or sports specific movements. There are several methods of stretching that are used for the purpose of increasing flexibility and include ballistic, static, dynamic and proprioceptive neuromuscular facilitation (PNF). Regardless of the method employed, it is important to remember that muscle tissue reduces in stiffness as the temperature of the muscle increases which supports the practice of performing a warm-up prior to stretching.

Ballistic stretching

With this particular method of stretching, muscles are taken to the end of their range of motion and then stretched further by bouncing movements. This method is usually performed by athletes as part of their training or competition routine. One of the drawbacks associated with ballistic stretching is that muscles are lengthened under force (and usually at speed) which can elicit a reflex action known as the 'stretch reflex' or 'myotatic reflex' which refers to a simple reflex action of the nervous system (no input from the brain) that operates in order to help maintain muscle tone and prevent injury. As shown in the example in figure 8.12 when a muscle is stretched both the muscle fibres (known as extrafusal fibres) and the muscle spindles (known as intrafusal fibres) lengthen. It is the muscle spindles that are responsible for initiating the reflex in response to muscles stretching

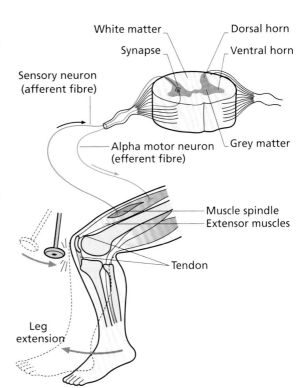

Figure 8.12 Example of the stretch reflex

which causes the muscle being stretched to contract. The faster the stretch the more forceful the contraction.

Static stretching

Static flexibility has been defined as 'the range of motion (ROM) available to a joint or a series of joints with no emphasis on speed during the stretch' whereas static stretching is 'stretching a muscle to a length just short of pain and maintaining that length for a period of time'. An increase in the range of motion following static stretching can be attributed to many factors but as yet, is not fully understood. There are varied suggestions as to how long a static (active or passive) stretch should be held to achieve the associated benefits. Research shows the same benefits from a static stretch lasting only a few seconds compared to stretches that last several minutes, therefore, the guidelines from the American college of Sports Medicine (ACSM) of 15–30 seconds duration are usually adopted. The trainer should make sure that static stretches are done slowly in order to minimise the effect of the stretch reflex. Static stretches can be categorised as either active or passive.

- **Passive stretching.** A passive stretch is a sub-classification of a static stretch and is considered to be when the individual makes no contribution to the generation of the stretching force (i.e. no voluntary muscular effort). An example of a passive stretch is a seated hamstring stretch where the individual leans forward with one leg outstretched. In passive stretching it is the weight of the body or gravity that is responsible for the stretch.
- **Active stretching.** This is a type of stretch that involves a voluntary contraction of a particular muscle to elicit a stretch of another muscle. For example, a concentric contraction of the tibialis anterior muscle would result in a stretch of the triceps surae (calf) muscle of the same leg. Active stretching is common among athletes, sports people and general fitness participants as it requires no participation of a partner or supervisor and once the technique has been demonstrated it can easily be learned and performed at any time by the individual.

Proprioceptive neuromuscular facilitation (PNF)

PNF stretching was initially used as a rehabilitation method for patients with cerebral palsy. This type of advanced stretching technique generally incorporates a static stretch of a target muscle followed by a short contraction (of that target muscle) against a resistance (normally a qualified partner). The target muscle is then again stretched further and the contraction against the resistance is repeated. The intensity of the contraction is difficult to estimate but low levels (in the region of 20–60% of maximum) of contraction intensity are generally recommended. This cycle of contraction and relaxation is usually repeated several times for one particular muscle group.

This type of stretching method is considered by many to produce greater and quicker gains in flexibility than those gains using static methods of stretching. Although the mechanisms of PNF are not fully understood, autogenic inhibition (previously known as the 'inverse myotatic reflex') and reciprocal inhibition are commonly cited as two of the main mechanisms involved in PNF stretching. It is the Golgi Tendon Organ (GTO) (a collection of specialist cells located in the musculo-tendinous junction) which responds to tension in the muscle whereby, if this becomes too great, the GTO inhibits muscle contraction causing the muscle to relax. It is thought that through regular PNF stretching, there is an alteration to the output from the muscle spindles and the Golgi Tendon Organs to the central nervous system, which results in increased flexibility. It is recommended that this type of stretching only be performed by those qualified to do so.

Dynamic stretching

This type of stretching is often associated with slow controlled rhythmic movements progressing through a full range of motion, depending on the muscle being stretched and the event being prepared for. Described as 'the ability to use a range of joint movement in the performance of a physical activity at normal or rapid speed' this type of flexibility is more applicable to sports or event-specific exercise as it involves movement.

Dynamic stretching exercises are normally carried out in a warm-up session and mimic the sport or event to follow. Not only do these exercises provide a rehearsal for the sporting or athletic events that are being prepared for, they also progressively raise the heart rate and mobilise specific joints. One of the mechanisms thought to be involved in dynamic flexibility is that of 'reciprocal inhibition'. When a muscle contracts (the agonist) the opposite (or antagonist) muscle relaxes to a certain degree. This occurs in order to allow the movement required by the contraction of the agonist muscle. If the antagonist muscle did not relax, the two muscles would be pulling against each other and no resultant movement would occur. Reciprocal inhibition (first described by Sherrington) is the term used to describe the amount of relaxation elicited in the antagonist muscle when the agonist muscle contracts. Regular dynamic stretching has been found to influence the amount of tension developed in the antagonist muscle during contraction of the agonist muscle. An example of reciprocal inhibition can be seen in figure 8.13. If the tension developed in the bicep brachii muscle and tricep brachii muscle is equal, then there will be no resultant movement. If the tension in the tricep brachii muscle reduces, the bicep brachii muscle will contract concentrically resulting in flexion at the elbow.

Because of the diverse nature of sport and exercise there are many dynamic stretching exercises that can be used effectively during warm-up sessions prior to main activity sessions. Table 8.11

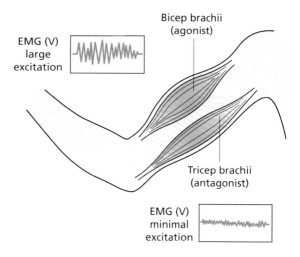

Figure 8.13 Example of reciprocal inhibition

provides a selection of exercises that trainers can choose from depending on the individual goals and nature of the client programme.

In terms of published guidelines on the performance of dynamic stretching exercises there is little consensus available, therefore, trainers should follow simple principles that are common to much of the literature. Many agree on the following:

1. Start slowly and progress to faster movements.
2. Contract the agonist muscle to stretch the antagonist muscle.
3. Start with small movements and gradually increase the range of motion.
4. End the intensity of the warm-up at the level required for the session to follow.
5. Incorporate whole body movements and mimic those that are specific to the sport or event.

Table 8.11	Common dynamic stretching exercises		
Name	**Baseline movement**	**Progression**	**Muscle stretched**
Balls of feet 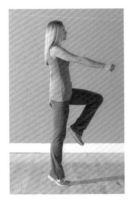	Rise up onto the balls of one foot and then lower. Alternate legs.	1. Walking toe raise. Roll from heel to toe while walking forward or back to achieve full extension of ankle. 2. Jogging slowly, point ankle (of the raised foot) at the floor in front.	Tibialis anterior
Straight legs 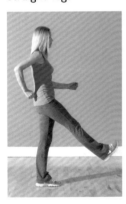	Fully extend the leg at a 45 degree angle and pull the toes back.	While walking, pull toes back on leading leg. At the same time, extend the heel maintaining a straight leg.	Calf (gastroc and soleus)
Knee hug 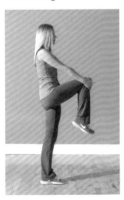	Pull alternate knee to chest in a controlled manner.	Walking, jogging then skipping, bringing knee to chest.	Gluteus maximus

Table 8.11	Common dynamic stretching exercises (*cont.*)		
Name	**Baseline movement**	**Progression**	**Muscle stretched**
Hamstring curl 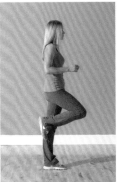	Bring heel to buttock with minimal hip flexion.	1. Bring the heel to the buttock during a staggered skip action. 2. Bring the heel to the buttock during a running action.	Quadriceps
Bowls stretch 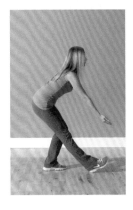	Put one foot about six inches in front of the other and pull the toes back. Bend from the waist and mimic a bowling action at the same time.	With leading leg straight and support leg bent, lean forward as if stretching the hamstring but keep walking forward and repeat with opposite leg.	Hamstrings
Lunge 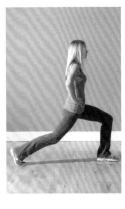	Adopt a lunge position.	With each stride adopt a lunge position on the move. Do the movements while travelling forwards and back.	Hip flexors

Table 8.11   Common dynamic stretching exercises (*cont.*)

Name	Baseline movement	Progression	Muscle stretched
Forward hurdle	Mimic the trailing leg of a hurdler as if going over a hurdle and then back.	Do the movements while travelling forwards and back.	Adductors
Knees across	Knees are raised high, and across the body.	Do the movements while travelling forwards and back.	Abductors
Arms across	Swing arms across the body at different angles.	This can be done on the spot and then while travelling.	Latissimus dorsi, trapezius, posterior deltoid

Table 8.11 Common dynamic stretching exercises (*cont.*)

Name	Baseline movement	Progression	Muscle stretched
Arms out 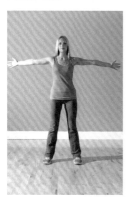	Swing the arms away from the body together at different angles.	This can be done on the spot and then while travelling.	Pectoralis major, anterior deltoid

MUSCULOSKELETAL SYSTEM

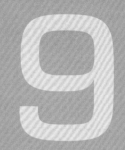

THE NOS LEVEL 3 PERSONAL TRAINER CRITERIA COVERED IN THIS CHAPTER ARE:

- The life-cycle of the musculoskeletal system (including bone) and its implications for working with young people, ante- and postnatal women, disabled people and older people (i.e. tendon, ligament and BMD changes and their effect on posture and postural stability for all the above)

SPECIAL POPULATIONS

One of the objectives of the screening process is to identify any client who would be categorised within a 'special population'. There is no universally accepted definition of the term 'special population' but it is often meant as a collective term for a group of people with specific health-related conditions that require a certain degree of expertise in relation to programme design and management over and above that required for an apparently 'healthy population'.

RELEVANT QUALIFICATIONS

The National Quality Assurance Framework, which was set up by the Department of Health in 2001, states that the minimum level of qualification recommended for exercise professionals, who are responsible for designing and delivering physical activity programmes for low- to medium-risk referred patients, is a level 3 advanced trainer award with a recognised exercise referral qualification. The range of potential medical conditions is extensive. Table 9.1 gives an overview of the conditions for which medical approval is considered (by the author) to be essential or whether it is just a recommendation. The table also gives an overview of the conditions for which specific qualifications are considered (by the author) to be essential for those supervising activity or whether they are just recommended.

L2 – Level 2 Trainer award
L3 – Level 3 advanced trainer award
L4 – Level 4 Specialist trainer award
BACR – British Association of Cardiac Rehabilitation (see chapter 12)

Table 9.1 Medical and qualification recommendations for all conditions

Condition	Medical approval		Specific qualification	
	Essential	Recommended	Essential	Recommended
Obesity		✓ (to identify any related condition)	✓ (L4)	
Diabetes	✓ (type 1)	✓ (type 2)	✓ (L4)	
COPD	✓			✓ (L3)
Asthma		✓		✓ (L3)
Hypertension	✓			✓ (L3)
Hyperlipidaemia		✓		✓ (L3)
Arthritis		✓		✓ (L3)
Osteoporosis		✓		✓ (L3)
Parkinson's		✓		✓ (L3)
Multiple sclerosis	✓			✓ (L3)
CVD	✓		✓ (BACR)	
Stroke	✓		✓ (BACR)	
Younger age			✓ (L2)	
Older age				✓ (L2)
Disability		✓		✓ (L2)
Ante- & postnatal		✓ (if currently inactive)	✓ (L2)	

Even though the range of special populations is diverse and recognised as such by SkillsActive, the national occupational standards refer specifically to the following populations:

- 14-16 year old young people
- older people (50+)
- ante- and postnatal women
- disabled people

Exercise has been shown to impact greatly on the musculoskeletal, cardiovascular and respiratory systems of those within these particular populations. It is important therefore that the trainer has a good working knowledge of the life-course of these systems (in particular the musculoskeletal system) and the implications for working with special population clients in terms of tendon, ligament and bone mass density (BMD) changes and their effect on posture and postural stability. It is also important that trainers understand the crucial aspect of pre-exercise screening and their role as a professional in dealing with clients of this nature.

SKELETAL DEVELOPMENT

The human skeleton, which is made up of 206 bones, consists of two parts: the axial skeleton (80 bones), which comprises the skull, vertebral column (backbone), ribs and sternum; and the appendicular skeleton (appendic meaning 'to hang on to') which comprises the shoulder and pelvic girdles and the upper and lower limbs. The shoulder or pectoral girdle attaches the arms to the body and consists of a scapula (shoulder blade) and clavicle (collar bone) on each side of the body. The scapula has a socket (glenoid fossa) or cavity, which joins with the upper arm (humerus) to form the shoulder joint. This is a shallow joint that allows for a large degree of mobility and therefore requires good muscle and ligament strength to contribute to stability. The pelvic girdle, on the other hand, provides a strong base in which the axial skeleton attaches via the vertebral column where it makes a fused joint with the sacrum. On each side of the pelvis there is a socket called the acetabulum, which forms a joint with the femur of the upper leg. The acetabulum is a deep socket that provides a high degree of stability but has less mobility than the shoulder joint. The pelvic girdle provides protection of internal organs and for a foetus during pregnancy.

GROWTH OF BONES

During growth development it is the long bones that grow in length at the region known as the 'epiphyseal' or 'growth plate'. This region is an area of cartilage near to the end of a long bone (see figure 9.1). The ends of a long bone are covered in a hard, shiny substance. This substance is known as 'articular cartilage', which is a very tough substance that helps to protect the ends of the bone. This is because it is the ends of bones that come together to form a joint where there will be movement, and as a result, friction would normally occur as the ends of the bone could actually rub against each other. Excessive exercise can cause this cartilage to wear down which could eventually lead to a condition known as 'arthritis'.

Bones do not grow at a steady rate throughout their life. The fastest rate of growth of bone is within the first two years of life when a child

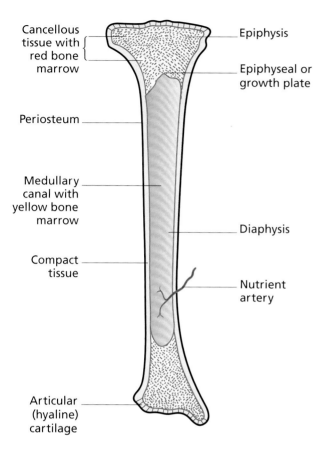

Cancellous tissue with red bone marrow

Periosteum

Medullary canal with yellow bone marrow

Compact tissue

Articular (hyaline) cartilage

Epiphysis

Epiphyseal or growth plate

Diaphysis

Nutrient artery

Figure 9.1 A typical long bone

not have the bone strength to cope with sustained high impact activities. Once the bones in the body stop growing, the growth plate area (which is made of cartilage during growth) is gradually replaced by bone.

Bone growth and the younger age

If normal growth occurs, it can reduce the chances of loss of bone mass and the likelihood of osteo-porosis (a condition in which bones weaken due to loss of mineral density) in later life. Regular physical activity into the mid-20s has been demonstrated to help develop bone mass with particular importance around the age of puberty. It has also been shown that weight-bearing activities such as jumping, dancing and aerobics, gymnastics, volleyball, racquet sports and football, etc., are particularly good for increasing bone mineral density. In general, the amount of physical activity that is needed for any kind of benefit appears to be achieved after only a few repetitions of an activity done on a regular basis. It has also been demonstrated that children who do these sorts of physical activities have, on average, 5–15% more bone mineral density than those children who are classed as inactive. According to a wide range of research, such as that by Boreham in 2001, having a higher bone mineral density is considered to significantly reduce the risk of osteoporotic fracture if the activities are maintained into older age (as long as the activities are done on a regular basis). Even though it is known that activity can have a positive effect on bone growth, too much exercise has been linked to certain injuries yet the exact amount, type and process is not completely understood. Bone injuries that are associated with excessive activity during childhood include chondromalacia patella and growth plate injuries.

can reach up to half of their full-grown height. Generally speaking, bone growth can continue until the early twenties at an average of about two inches a year but girls generally mature physiologically about 2–2.5 years earlier than boys do. Growth spurts tend to occur at different times in life for boys and girls. For girls, the main growth spurt typically occurs between the age of 10 and 13 years. For boys, growth spurts typically occur around the age of 12–14 years. As bones are still growing at this age, this often means that children are more susceptible to certain injuries as they do

- **Chondromalacia patella** (also known as runner's knee). Female hips are generally wider than male hips. Wide hips result in the femur (the upper leg bone) being placed at a greater inward angle than is normal. This can cause injury to the patella, which occurs when the patella does not run smoothly in the groove at the end of the femur. In this situation the cartilage on the back of the patella can wear away, causing pain.
- **Growth plate injuries.** As mentioned earlier, bone growth occurs near the ends of long bones (epiphyseal or growth plate) so that the bone grows in length. Excessive loads at the area of the growth plate can sometimes negatively affect bone growth.

Effects of ageing on the skeletal system

There are many reported changes associated with ageing and the skeletal system. Main changes include:

- decreased bone mineral content and increased fracture risk
- long-term stress on joints
- decreased availability of synovial fluid/calcification of cartilage
- reduced joint stability and range of movement
- thinned intervertebral discs
- associated postural and postural stability problems

A reduction in bone strength (due to a decrease in bone mineral density) is a major ageing change that can result in disorders that are common among elderly people such as osteoporosis and postural problems. Loss of bone mass over the years (known as osteoporosis) can substantially increase the risk of fractures from falls, therefore, it is crucial that regular physical activity is maintained in order to help to slow down bone mass loss and maintain a good level of balance, which should help prevent falls. Even though bone strength does not continue to increase once adulthood has arrived (although there is a thought that some gain is still possible), it is important to slow down the rate of bone loss. Physical activity, especially strength training, can be of benefit for all ages, although old bone responds more slowly than young bone. Also, because of the amount of movement that has taken place over the years, the joints and associated structures often suffer as a result. This can manifest in conditions such as osteoarthritis and stiffness, especially in areas such as the spine and hips which can lead to quite severe postural problems.

MUSCULAR DEVELOPMENT

When discussing the development of muscle tissue within the body it is useful to have a general understanding of the composition and roles of the different types of fibres relating to what we know as 'skeletal muscle'.

MUSCLE TYPES

There are actually three types of muscle tissue that can be found in the human body:

- Cardiac muscle – the heart muscle
- Smooth muscle – for squeezing (peristaltic) action, e.g. digestive system
- Skeletal muscle – for movement. Mainly attached to bones

Each type of muscle within the body develops throughout childhood. For instance, the heart

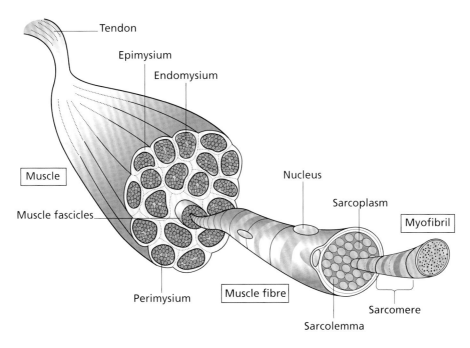

Figure 9.2 A typical skeletal muscle structure

becomes larger and stronger in order to pump a greater volume of blood around a larger body. Smooth muscle in the digestive system and other places such as the arteries also develops its contraction ability in order to squeeze contents through the intestine and arteries, such as food and blood.

Skeletal muscle

Muscles are made up of individual muscle fibres (made up of proteins) which run the entire length of the muscle. These fibres are called 'myofibrils' as can be seen in figure 9.2.

In some muscles there might only be relatively few fibres such as in muscles of the eye in which there are only tens of fibres. In some of the bigger muscles in the body there may be thousands of fibres. For instance, there can be up to 400,000 fibres in the bicep muscle which is in the front of the arm. Each muscle fibre is surrounded by a sheath of fibrous tissue membrane or fascia (meaning bandage) called endomysium (endo-, meaning within). This can be envisaged as a sausage wrapped in a skin. Muscle fibres are then grouped together in a bundle (fascicle) and surrounded by another fascia sheath called perimysium (peri-, meaning around). Finally, another fascia sheath called epimysium (epi-, meaning upon) surrounds the entire muscle. At each end of the muscle the three types of fascia sheath taper off and converge together to form an attachment to the bone. The attachment point of muscle to bone is called 'tendon' and when muscle contracts it pulls on the tendon, which in turn pulls on the bone and causes movement. Skeletal muscles are known as 'voluntary' as they require conscious thought for movement to occur as opposed to movement being automatic (except in the case of a reflex). About 40–46% of body weight between the ages of 5 and 29 years is made up of muscle tissue. The largest muscle in the body is the gluteus maximus, which is the main part of the buttock. The strongest muscle is usually considered to be the quadricep (front of the thigh), even though the jaw can create a greater force. The longest muscle in the body is the sartorious running from the iliac spine in the pelvis to the medial aspect of the tibia (top of the shin).

Fibre types

There are many different types of skeletal muscle fibres but they are commonly split into two groups: slow and fast twitch. Slow twitch fibres are also known as Type I fibres and fast twitch fibres are further split in to Type IIa and Type IIb fibres. The differences in the fibres can be seen in table 9.2.

Human beings have different percentages of all three fibre types in each muscle group depending on their genetics. It is possible to change the way fibres behave but only by a small amount as 'we are what we were born with', and training can only have a small, if sometimes crucial, effect. As with skeletal growth, the muscles in the body also grow at irregular rates.

The enlargement of muscles (known as 'hyper-trophy') makes them thicker but muscle fibres can also get longer. At puberty, boys tend to have a faster rate of muscle growth than girls due to increased levels of testosterone, which helps to build muscles. With certain types of training and genetics, boys' muscle mass can peak at about 50% of body weight around the age of 18 to 25 years, whereas girls' muscle mass peaks at about 40% of body weight around the age of 16 to 20 years.

Table 9.2	Common characteristics of muscle fibres		
	Type I	**Type IIA**	**Type II B**
Contraction time	Slow	Fast	Very Fast
Resistance to fatigue	High	Intermediate	Low
Activity used for	Aerobic	Longer-term anaerobic	Short-term anaerobic
Force production	Low	High	Very high
Colour	Reddish	Whitish	Whitish
Blood supply	Very good	Not as good	Not so good
Main fuel	Fat	Carbohydrate	Carbohydrate

Effects of ageing on the muscular system

As with the skeletal system there are many reported changes associated with ageing and the muscular system. Main changes include:

- reduced motor function (reduced motor unit size and loss of fine control)
- decreased size and number of muscle fibres
- fewer fast twitch fibres
- reduced concentration of protein
- reduced size and number of mitochondria
- reduced capillarity
- increased connective tissue
- reduced strength and power

The heart is not the only muscle in the body that can weaken with age, as a reduction in muscular strength and power is also evident within the older population. This has been demonstrated in studies such as that by Skelton *et al* in 1995, whereby there is a general agreement that muscle strength decreases at a rate of about 10% per decade up to as much as 60% total loss by the age of 80. This reduction can have a negative effect on the daily lives of older people in that they will not be able, or will find it difficult, to perform tasks they once found relatively easy. The loss of muscle mass that occurs with age (known as sarcopenia) is one of the main causes of weakness and lack of mobility. Other causes include the reduction in motor unit size and a decrease in size and number of muscle fibres (especially fast twitch which are capable of the greatest force).

Certain types of physical activity have been shown to help slow down the loss of muscle mass, but it cannot stop or reverse the process. Even though the cause of muscle mass loss is not fully understood, it is quite clear that ageing is the main cause and, according to studies such as that by Roubenoff and Hughes in 2000, inactivity can speed up this process. It is important to understand that physical activity needs to continue into old age as, according to studies such as that by Benvenuti *et al* in 2000, physical activity levels up to middle age have no effect on muscle strength in old age. Another problem is that when older people stop doing regular physical activity, the loss of muscle mass and strength occurs faster than it does during youth and middle age. This is a huge problem as loss of muscle strength can increase the risk of osteoporosis and falls which in turn increases the risk of bone fracture and, as shown in studies such as that by Chu *et al* in 1999, muscle weakness in the legs is linked to the number of falls. Therefore, regular strength training for older adults using external weights or body weight resistance exercises should not be underestimated as it has been shown to be highly effective in increasing or just maintaining muscle strength, even into very old age (Narici 2000). Not only do muscles lose strength and power but they also lose elasticity, which means that flexibility can also be lost. Flexibility is further affected by cartilage surrounding joints calcifying which leads to a decrease in the range of motion at the joint. Because of the loss of muscle strength (and muscle mass) and reduction in flexibility, older people tend not to be as active, which leads to an increase of adipose tissue and hence fat percentage.

LIGAMENT DEVELOPMENT

Made of collagen, ligaments are tough, white, non-elastic fibrous tissues strung together in a strap-like formation. They are attached from bone to bone allowing wanted movement and preventing unwanted movement. Many ligaments are present at birth and develop over the lifetime of the individual. As ligaments have limited stretch capability, any excessive stretching can cause tears and in some cases complete rupture. The healing time of ligament tissue with a partial tear is relatively slow due to the poor blood supply and depending on the severity of the damage to the ligament it can take weeks to months for the healing process to complete.

Trainers should be aware that ligament injuries are often left untreated and as such compromise the stability of the relevant joint and in cases that affect the ankle, balance ability is usually decreased. Trainers should always try and identify previous ligament injuries during screening and make any considerations necessary in their programming as ligaments can become stronger and in some cases hypertrophy (become larger) following weight-bearing activities, and balance ability can also be improved even into older age. It should be noted however that ligaments (and tendons) tend to lose their elasticity during ageing, therefore, stability can be compromised.

TENDON DEVELOPMENT

Tendons are bluish-white slightly elastic fascia tissue which connect muscles to bone. They are made up of the sheaths that surround the muscle fibres and attach to the periostium covering on the bone. In some cases the area of connection is relatively small, as in the bicep brachii tendons, but in other cases the tendon can be spread out in sheets over a wide area, as in the tibialis anterior. These spread out tendon attachments are called aponeuroses. When muscles contract they pull from the middle and exert a pulling force on the tendons at each end of the muscle (origin and insertion). As the tendons are connected to bone they will attempt to pull the bones together. If one of the bones remains in a fixed position, the other bone will move towards it and create movement. Tendons stretch only slightly but not as much as muscle tissue and prolonged tension on tendon tissue may result in tearing. They are reasonably slow to heal as the blood supply to tendons is less than that to muscles. As in the case of ligaments, tendons will also become stronger with weight-bearing activity. It is also possible in the case of extreme force for the tendon to pull away from the attachment point at the periostium (this is called an avulsion). This can be a partial tear where there is still some tendon attached or a complete rupture where the entire tendon is torn from the periostium. If this occurs, the muscle will have no attachment at one end and, therefore, will be unable to move the bones it is attached to. This often requires surgery, whereas a partial tear can heal in time. Tendons can also become inflamed through repetitive use. This type of injury is known as tendonitis (-itis means inflammation). There are common tendon injuries that are associated with both younger and older age groups. In the case of younger age groups typical injuries include:

- **Osgood-Schlatter disease** (See http://www.patient.co.uk/health/Osgood-Schlatter's-Disease.htm). This is the name of a common condition in which the patella (knee cap) tendon pulls away from its attachment point just below the knee (the tibial tuberosity). It is usually caused as a result of excessive impact over a period of time, which eventually results in a build-up of scar tissue that subsequently causes pain.

Table 9.3 Cardiovascular and respiratory differences between special populations

Special population group	Main cardiovascular differences	Exercise implication
Children/young people	• Walking/running economy is less. • Cardiac output and stroke volume lower. • Thermoregulation not as efficient. • Higher maximum heart rate.	• Perform extended warm-up/cool-downs and limit duration of higher intensity activities. Avoid extremes of temperature and keep well hydrated, especially in winter. Always supervise exercises.
Older adults	• Cardiac output, stroke volume, VO_2max and heart rate decrease. • Blood pressure increases. • Capillaries decrease in number.	• Any progression should be slow and to individual capacity. Get regular feedback during and after exercise. Introduce post-exercise relaxation. Avoid fatigue. Use cycling and swimming for those with reduced weight-bearing capacity.
Ante/postnatal	• Increase in resting heart rate. • Decrease in venous return. • Cardiac output increases. • Left ventricle and blood vessels enlarge. • Blood flow to the skin increases.	• Avoid motionless or exercise in the supine position. Be aware of heating up quickly. Limit higher intensity to short periods. No high impact and no exhaustion. Low intensity only (after medical approval) if there is no history of exercise. Stop if any pain or discomfort.
Children/young people	• Higher breathing rate (ventilation).	• Children have to breathe faster for any given intensity so reduce the duration of high intensity exercise.
Older adults	• Lung capacity and forced expiratory volume decrease due to muscle weakness and loss of alveoli elasticity. Maximal ventilation decreases.	• Reduce intensity of exercise due to shortness of breath. Work on back muscle strength as posture becomes worse.
Ante/postnatal	• Higher breathing rate (ventilation) as a result of increased sensitivity to carbon dioxide. • Decreased residual volume. • Increased oxygen consumption. • Hyperventilation can occur.	• Reduce intensity of exercise due to shortness of breath (even at low intensity). Be aware that hyperventilation can occur.

- **Sever's disease.** When the Achilles tendon (this is the tendon at the back of the lower leg running into the heel bone) repetitively pulls on its attachment point at the heel it can also cause pain just like the patella tendon. The Achilles tendon was named after the Greek hero Achilles in the Trojan War. It was thought that his only weak point was his heel and so to this day someone's weak point is referred to as their Achilles heel.

In the case of older groups, injuries tend to be of a repetitive-type nature known as Repetitive Strain Injury (RSI). Two of the most common that the trainer may have to deal with are 'tennis elbow' and 'golfer's elbow'.

- **Tennis elbow.** The condition 'lateral epicondylitis' is often referred to colloquially as tennis elbow (and sometimes shooter's elbow or archer's elbow). It is a condition where the bony outer part of the elbow (the lateral epicondyle) becomes sore and tender as a result of overuse of the posterior muscles in the forearm. Twisting and gripping movements tend to be the cause of the condition, therefore, trainers should try to eliminate any unnecessary twisting during execution of resistance exercises. For example, during the bicep curl start with the hands in the anatomical position (arms hanging by the side and the palms facing forward) rather than facing inwards which requires a twist.

- **Golfer's elbow.** The condition 'medial epicondylitis' is often referred to colloquially as golfer's elbow (and sometimes pitcher's elbow or climber's elbow). It is a condition where the bony inner part of the elbow (the medial epicondyle) becomes sore and tender as a result of overuse of the anterior muscles in the forearm. As grip tension is cited as a main cause, trainers should constantly reinforce clients to loosen the grip if they feel it is too tight.

CARDIOVASCULAR AND RESPIRATORY SYSTEM CHANGES

There are many changes associated with the cardiovascular and respiratory systems in special population groups. Although beyond the scope of this book it is important for trainers to take these effects into consideration as described in table 9.3.

EXERCISE GUIDELINES

THE NOS LEVEL 3 PERSONAL TRAINER CRITERIA COVERED IN THIS CHAPTER ARE:

- The life-cycle of the musculoskeletal system (including bone) and its implications for working with young people, ante- and postnatal women, disabled people and older people (i.e. tendon, ligament and BMD changes and their effect on posture and postural stability for all the above)
- Contraindications and key safety guidelines for working with older clients
- Contraindications and key safety guidelines for working with ante- and postnatal clients
- How to give guidance to encourage special population clients to follow the key safety guidelines and to discourage them from anything deemed to be potentially hazardous/contraindicated to enable them to take part in sessions

EXERCISE GUIDELINES FOR YOUNGER AND OLDER AGE GROUPS

Many of the published physical activity guidelines related to special populations differ depending on the source. As with guidelines for the apparently healthy population, those from the American College of Sports Medicine (ACSM) tend to be widely adopted across the UK health and fitness industry, which results in a consistency of delivery by trainers. It is interesting however to compare against credible sources within the UK such as the Department of Health. With respect to the intensity, duration and frequency of physical activity,

table 10.1 gives an overview of the ACSM's physical activity guidelines for children over the age of 5 years up to the age of 16 years.

It is interesting to note that according to the Department of Health (2004), one hour of physical activity each day may not be enough to prevent the current rising obesity trends that can be seen in children but may have important health benefits with respect to other diseases. The DoH recommends therefore, that children and young people should achieve a total of at least 60 minutes of moderate intensity (equivalent to brisk walking which might leave the participant feeling warm and slightly out of breath) physical activity each day. They also recommend that at least twice a week this should include activities to improve bone health, muscle strength and flexibility. Trainers should be aware that it is difficult to estimate the intensity at which children are exercising therefore it is advised to use the modified version of the Borg Rating of Perceived Exertion Scale for children (see figure 10.1). As with adults, the scale is shown to children during the activities they are doing and they

Table 10.1	ACSM physical activity guidelines for older children	
	Aerobic Training	**Strength Training**
MODE	• Any kind of activity that includes weight bearing	• Body weight and bands may be required before progressing to weights
INTENSITY	• Moderate to vigorous intensity • Choose activities that are intermittent in nature • Emphasise active play rather than exercise for younger children	• Use 8–15RM • Overload by increasing repetitions then intensity
DURATION	• 20–30 minutes per session • 30–60 for overweight and obese	• Perform 1 or 2 sets of 8–10 different exercises • 1–2 minutes rest between exercises
FREQUENCY	• At least 3 days per week • 6–7 days for overweight and obese	• 2 sessions per week • Encourage other forms of exercise
PRECAUTIONS	• Be aware of children overheating quickly	• Balance upper and lower body • Overload by increasing repetitions then intensity • Avoid muscular fatigue

GENERAL PRECAUTIONS:
• All activities should be supervised
• Learn technique before strength
• Perform full range multi-joint exercises if possible
• Avoid any ballistic movements
• Perform extended warm-up / cool-downs
• Avoid mismatching sizes when pairing/grouping children together
• If the temperature exceeds 30°C, children should not exercise for longer than 20 minutes and should be well hydrated before, during and after activities
• If the temperature exceeds 38°C (100°F), children should not exercise outside
• It is important for children (and adults) to drink water before, during and after any activity

Intensity	Explanation
0-rest	How you feel when sitting or resting
1-easy	Light walking; not sweating
2-pretty hard	Playing in the playground and just starting to sweat
3-harder	Playing hard and sweating
4-hard	Running around hard and sweating a lot
5-maximal	Hardest you have ever worked, ready to collapse

Figure 10.1 Adapted modified version of Borg's RPE scale for children

are asked to estimate what level they think they are exercising at.

For older age groups the aims of a physical activity programme should be to reduce the physical deterioration and social dysfunction of older individuals. Emphasis should be placed on the improvement of ability with respect to the performance of everyday activities (known as Functions for Daily Living or FDLs) as there are many positive benefits of regular physical activity.

FUNCTION FOR DAILY LIVING

When talking about the elderly, it is quite common for research to talk in terms of Activities of Daily Living (ADL) and Instrumental Activities of Daily Living (IADL) (see table 10.2). It is not surprising to know that the ability to perform ADL and IADL decreases with age. Generally speaking, more than one-third of the UK elderly

population will have ADL or IADL problems resulting from chronic health conditions such as arthritis, heart disease and diabetes.

Although the trainer should focus on functions for daily living in terms of short-, medium- or long-term goals, there are many gym-based exercises (as there are for apparently healthy populations) that can help to achieve these goals. With respect to the intensity, duration and frequency of physical activity, table 10.3 gives an overview of the ACSM's physical activity guidelines for older adults.

As with guidelines for children it is interesting to compare the ACSM guidelines for older adults with those of the Department of Health (DoH). As can be seen in table 10.4, guidelines are similar with the main difference relating to the reference of sedentary activity as mentioned by the Department of Health.

There are few absolute contraindications for exercise by older adults; however, there are some that have been suggested such as unstable coronary artery disease or recent myocardial infarction (heart attack), congestive heart failure that has progressed to dyspnoea (breathlessness) at rest,

Table 10.2 Common ADL and IADL	
Activities of daily living (ADL)	Instrumental activities of daily living (IADL)
• Bathing	• Cooking
• Eating	• Shopping
• Dressing	• Managing money
• Toilet duties	• Using the telephone
• Getting around	• Doing housework
	• Taking medication

Table 10.3 ACSM physical activity guidelines for sedentary older adults

	Aerobic Training	Strength Training
MODE	• Walking, cycling and water-based activities are better for those with reduced tolerance for weight bearing.	• Body weight and bands may be required before progressing to weights.
INTENSITY	• Work to individual capacity.	• Overload by increasing repetitions before intensity.
DURATION	• 20–30 minutes per session. • Increase duration rather than intensity. Slow progression.	• Perform 2 to 3 sets of 12–15RM. • 1–2 minutes rest between exercises.
FREQUENCY	• 3-5 days per week.	• 2–3 sessions per week. • Encourage other forms of exercise.
PRECAUTIONS	• Constantly monitor feedback and use RPE scales.	• Avoid muscular fatigue. • Balance upper and lower body.

GENERAL PRECAUTIONS:
• Be wary when setting goals as progression is often slow.
• Get feedback relating to muscle soreness especially if the individual is inexperienced.
• Relaxation is recommended post-exercise.
• Take into consideration any condition the individual may have.

tachyarrhythmia (irregular fast heart rate) induced by activity, and critical aortic stenosis (narrowing of the aorta). Non-cardiac contraindications suggested include the immediate hypoxic period after pulmonary emboli (lung blockage leading to lack of oxygen), retinal detachment, and unstable cervical spinal conditions.

Conditions such as these should have been identified during the screening session with the client. Should the trainer feel that they are not qualified in any way to deal with an identified condition then they should refer the client to their own GP in order to clarify the situation and if necessary gain the consent of the GP.

ANTE- AND POSTNATAL CONSIDERATIONS

There are many complications and factors to take into consideration during pregnancy so trainers should undertake a specialist qualification in this area if they feel that this population will be featuring in their client base. For those who may only work occasionally with this population it is worth considering three main effects of pregnancy: hormone release, diastasis recti and pelvic girdle pain.

HORMONE RELEASE

One of the main effects during pregnancy (and lasts for a period of months afterwards) is the

Table 10.4	DoH physical activity guidelines for older adults

1   Older adults who participate in any amount of physical activity gain some health benefits, including maintenance of good physical and cognitive function. Some physical activity is better than none, and more physical activity provides greater health benefits.

2   Older adults should aim to be active daily. Over a week, activity should add up to at least 150 minutes (2½ hours) of moderate intensity activity in bouts of 10 minutes or more – one way to approach this is to do 30 minutes at least 5 days a week.

3   For those who are already regularly active at moderate intensity, comparable benefits can be achieved through 75 minutes of vigorous intensity activity spread across the week or a combination of moderate and vigorous activity.

4   Older adults should also undertake physical activity to improve muscle strength on at least two days a week.

5   Older adults at risk of falls should incorporate physical activity to improve balance and coordination on at least two days a week.

6   All older adults should minimise the amount of time spent being sedentary (sitting) for extended periods.

release of hormones, in particular one known as relaxin, which is produced initially by the ovaries, and then by the placenta later in pregnancy. Although the exact mechanism is still under investigation, it is thought that relaxin affects the collagen fibres of all connective tissue in the body making ligaments and tendons more pliable and joints less stable, especially the sacro-iliac joint and pubic symphysis. The main change in relation to posture comes as a result of the body having to adapt to the change in the centre of gravity, which moves outwards and also slightly down. As a result of this shift in the centre of gravity, there are several negative postural effects that can occur, which can eventually lead to back pain in many cases. These postural effects include:

- Lengthening and weakening of abdominal muscles
- Ligaments loosen mainly around the hips, lower back and pelvis
- As a result of weakened muscles there is reduced support for the spine
- This weakness also causes an increased lumbar lordosis (hollow lower back) and an increased thoracic kyphosis (rounded upper back)
- The pelvis can also tilt forward which also increases the lumbar curve

A pregnant woman typically displays a different pattern of gait. The step or stride lengthens as the pregnancy progresses, as a result of the weight gain and changes in posture. The combined effect of an increase in body weight during pregnancy, fluid retention, and weight gain, lowers the arches of the foot adding to the foot's length and width which may result in the typical 'waddling' gait seen in many pregnant women.

DIASTASIS RECTI

One of the main abdominal muscles that is often affected by pregnancy is the rectus abdominis, which lengthens and becomes wider. When this occurs the muscle might appear to split down the middle as can be seen in figure 10.2 but it is actually a band of tendon (or aponeurosis) called the 'linea alba', which separates to allow for growth of the baby and swelling of the abdomen area. This separation of the rectus abdominis muscle is known as 'diastasis recti' and occurs in about two-thirds of all pregnant women.

PELVIC GIRDLE PAIN

During pregnancy the sacroiliac (the joint between the sacrum and the illium) and sacrococcygeal (the joint between the sacrum and the coccyx) joints become loose to allow the symphysis pubis to widen for birth. Excessive widening can compromise the stability of the pelvic girdle (and can also affect pelvic stability after delivery) and can lead to pain in the lower back, the pubic area and down into the legs, where it may be mistaken for sciatica. This is referred to as 'pregnancy-related pelvic girdle pain' (PGP) and although relatively common (experienced by up to 45% of pregnant women) it is not considered to be 'normal' as it can lead to problems with walking, everyday activities and weight-bearing on one leg.

Almost any movements of the hips can cause discomfort or pain so it is important to try and minimise this discomfort by keeping the hips aligned and stable. Taking shorter walking strides, avoiding crossing the legs or adduction at the hip, keeping activity low-impact and short duration are all strategies that can all help to minimise the pain. Trainers working with clients who suspect they suffer from PGP must refer them to their GP for

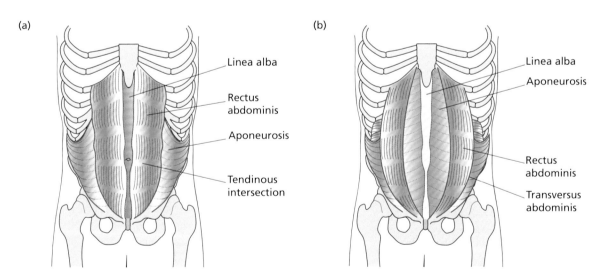

(a)

Linea alba

Rectus abdominis

Aponeurosis

Tendinous intersection

(b)

Linea alba

Aponeurosis

Rectus abdominis

Transversus abdominis

Figure 10.2 Abdominal wall before and after diastasis recti

clinical investigation before undertaking further exercise. If consent for exercise is given, the trainer must ensure the pelvis is correctly aligned during any exercise in order to avoid exacerbating the condition. As far as general guidelines for antenatal physical activity are concerned, table 10.5 provides an overview taken from a variety of sources such as the RCOG, the ACOG and the American College of Sports Medicine. Note that activity should only be progressed between the 13th and 28th weeks.

Table 10.5 Physical activity guidelines for Antenatal women		
	Aerobic Training	**Strength Training**
MODE	• Walking, cycling and water-based activities are good for this condition.	• Continue as normal if already active. If not, slow progression from body weight to machines/free-weights.
INTENSITY	• RPE level 10–14 • 60-80% HRmax	• Avoid heavy loads. • Overload by increasing repetitions.
DURATION	• 5–45 minutes per session. • Increase by 2 mins per week but only between the 13th and 28th weeks.	• Perform 1 to 3 sets of 15-20RM. • 1–2 minutes rest between exercises.
FREQUENCY	Active person: • 3-4 per week up to 14th week • 3-5 per week up to 28th week • 3 per week after 28th week Non-active person: • None before 13th week • 3 per week 13th-36th weeks • 1–2 per week after 36th week	• 2–3 sessions per week. • Encourage other forms of exercise. • Decrease weight and sets and increase recovery time as pregnancy progresses.
PRECAUTIONS	• Avoid high-impact activities and excessive repetition. • Watch for signs of overheating.	• If no experience prior to pregnancy, do not start. • Avoid overstretching and overhead lifts.

GENERAL PRECAUTIONS:
• Non-active women are advised to seek medical approval before beginning a programme of activity
• If any activity causes pain or discomfort, it should be stopped immediately.
• Do rectus abdominis check 6–12 weeks after delivery before doing certain abdominal exercises.
• Be aware of episiotomy and take appropriate steps.
• Avoid motionless standing.
• Avoid supine exercises (lying on the back) after 16 weeks.

Due to the nature of the condition, there are many reasons why a pregnant individual should not take part in an exercise session (known as contraindications). Even though some of these terms may be unfamiliar, trainers should ask clients during screening if they have any of the contraindications and refer to a GP for advice and consent if they do. It is important also that

Table 10.6	Contraindications and reasons to stop activity for pregnant women (RCOG)

Absolute contraindications to activity

- Haemodynamically significant heart disease
- Restrictive lung disease
- Incompetent cervix/cerclage
- Multiple gestation at risk of preterm labour
- Persistent bleeding in the second and third trimesters
- Placenta praevia after 26 weeks
- Pre-eclampsia or pregnancy-induced hypertension
- Preterm labour (previous/present)
- Preterm rupture of membranes

Relative contraindications to activity

- Severe anaemia (haemoglobin less than 100 g/l)
- Unevaluated maternal cardiac arrhythmia
- Chronic bronchitis
- Poorly controlled type 1 diabetes
- Extreme morbid obesity ((BMI > 40)
- Extreme underweight (BMI <12)
- Extremely sedentary lifestyle
- Intrauterine growth restriction in current pregnancy
- Poorly controlled hypertension/pre-eclampsia
- Orthopaedic limitations
- Poorly controlled thyroid disease
- Poorly controlled seizure disorder
- Heavy smoker (more than 20 cigarettes/day)

Reasons to stop activity

- Excessive shortness of breath
- Chest pain or palpitations
- Presyncope or dizziness
- Painful uterine contractions or preterm labour
- Calf pain or swelling
- Leakage of amniotic fluid
- Vaginal bleeding
- Excessive fatigue
- Abdominal pain, particularly in back or pubic area
- Pelvic girdle pain
- Reduced foetal movement
- Dyspnoea before exertion
- Headache or visual disturbance
- Muscle weakness
- Sudden calf pain or swelling in the ankles, hands or face
- Insufficient weight gain (less than 1 kg per month) – during last two trimesters

the trainer constantly monitor exercise sessions for circumstances that require the activity to be stopped immediately (as in table 10.6 as suggested by the RCOG).

DISABILITY

The term 'disability' is difficult to describe and is often misunderstood. This is because the definition could be based on a medical model or a social model, or another model entirely. In the case of the medical model, an individual can be born with a so-called disability such as Down's syndrome or cerebral palsy, or they could acquire a disability through an illness, chronic disease or as a result of an injury. Also within the medical model there could be mental health problems such as depression, dementia and schizophrenia, which are commonly thought of as disabilities. However, some definitions refer to a social model of disability and how some people do not 'fit in' and are therefore considered to be disabled.

Regardless of the definition, disability can vary widely in terms of type, severity and duration (refer to the WHO 2000 for classifications of disability). For example, disabilities can affect a person's ability to walk, see, hear, understand or speak. Because of this extreme variation, it is important to understand that every disability is different and even the same type or category of disability can affect each individual differently. It is better, therefore, to focus less on the definition of disability and to think in terms of what disabled people can do rather than any restrictions that they might have relating to a particular condition. According to the English Federation of Disability Sport there are between 8 and 12 million people in the UK with some degree of disability or impairment as defined as Disabled under the Disability Discrimination Act (DDA). The Disability Discrimination Act of 2005 provides guidance on the acts and regulations relating to the provision of exercise and physical activity.

INCLUSION

The use of the term inclusion is becoming more widespread, especially in schools, sports clubs and exercise environments. This particular term simply means to create environments that are accessible, safe and supportive of persons of all ages, gender and abilities. There are many barriers that are experienced by people with disabilities that cannot be seen, such as negative attitudes of others, lack of knowledge or situations where communication is difficult. Barriers such as these should never be allowed to exist as there are many simple things that can be done to ensure that all individuals are given the same opportunities to participate in physical activity. Simple solutions, such as providing necessary adaptive equipment (including accessible fitness, sports or recreation equipment) to allow individuals with disabilities to participate fully, are easy to put in place. It can also help if those delivering sessions know how to use specialised equipment and how to adapt activities for different disabilities.

TERMINOLOGY

People are often confused about what they think is the correct terminology to use when relating to disability. The attempt to be 'politically correct' can often create confusion and embarrassing situations, therefore, it is recommended that if people are unsure about the terminology to use then an easy solution to this is simply asking the person with the disability what words they would prefer to be used. Table 10.7 gives an overview of some of the current terms that are used in relation to various disabilities. It must be mentioned however, that these terms can change in their 'political correctness' so it is always recommended that trainers visit the website of the leading body related to each disability category for up-to-date information.

Table 10.7	Common terms related to disability
Term	**Description**
Disability	General term used for a functional limitation that interferes with a person's ability and can be a physical, sensory or mental condition.
Non-disabled	This was previously able-bodied.
Handicap	A physical or attitudinal constraint imposed upon a person, regardless of whether or not that person has a disability.
Hemiplegia	Full or partial paralysis of one side of the body.
Paraplegia	Paralysis of the lower half of the body including the partial or total loss of function of both legs.
Quadriplegia	Paralysis of the body involving partial or total loss of function in both arms and legs.
Down's syndrome	A chromosome disorder that usually causes a delay in physical, intellectual and language development. Usually results in mental retardation. Joints can also be unstable due to lax ligaments.
Hearing impairment	Refers to partial or total loss of auditory functioning. Do not refer to 'the deaf' but instead say 'people who are deaf'.
Speech impairment	Some level of speech problem that causes speaking difficulty.
Cerebral palsy	Brain lesions leading to movement and speech problems. Not called spasticity any more.
Additional needs	Used to be called special needs.
Learning disability	A group of neurological conditions (e.g. dyslexia, dysgraphia, dyscalculia) which affect the person's ability to receive, interpret and use information.
Mental disability	Psychiatric disability, retardation, learning disability and cognitive impairment.
Muscular dystrophy	A condition that affects muscle fibres and causes weakness. Often results in the use of a powered wheelchair.

Table 10.8 Common misconceptions related to disability

Misconception	Reality
Having a disability means that you are not or cannot be healthy.	People with disabilities can achieve good health as they can benefit from healthy activities as much as the general population.
Wheelchair use implies that users of wheelchairs are 'wheelchair-bound'.	A wheelchair, much the same as a bicycle, is just a device that helps someone to get around.
You shouldn't ask people about their disabilities.	Most people with disabilities won't mind answering your questions.
People with disabilities always need help.	Many people with disabilities are quite independent but if you want to help, then just ask them if they need any.

It is an unfortunate fact that in today's society there are many misconceptions about individuals with disabilities. Many of these misconceptions are not based on evidence, rather a lack of understanding or ignorance is the main problem. Even as recently as 20 or 30 years ago, there was limited access for the public regarding information related to specific disabilities. In today's society, however, this is just not the case as the information available is vast and easily accessible. Table 10.8 gives an overview of some of the most common misconceptions that people have about those with disabilities and what the reality associated with it generally is.

BENEFITS OF PHYSICAL ACTIVITY

Individuals with disabilities are often less active than those without disabilities, yet they are at risk of the same health problems as well as problems related to their disability such as fatigue, obesity, lack of self-esteem, social exclusion, etc. There is a wealth of evidence to show that participation in physical activity for those with a disability can lead to improved levels of both physical health and psychological well-being (such as self-confidence, social awareness and self-esteem). In other words, physical activity can play an important role in the lives of those with disabilities, the same as it can for those without disabilities.

Before beginning any programme of physical activity, however, it is always a good idea to consult with the disabled individual to highlight any restrictions there may be. In terms of those people with physical disabilities, the benefits of physical activity are almost identical to those for non-disabled people, taking into account the specific impact of the disability. In terms of mental health problems, according to the English Federation of Disability Sport, they are now the UK's highest cause of time off work, with nearly three out of ten employees suffering a stress- or mental-health-related problem every year. This is quite an important statistic considering that about 21% of people with a mental health condition are in employment and that the World Health Organization estimates that by 2020 depression will become the second most important cause of disability in the world. Even though the effects of physical activity on mental health conditions are not fully understood, it is generally thought that there will be a beneficial effect in most cases. This supports the view by the American College of Sports Medicine that depression often accompanies a disability but can be improved by physical activity.

INTERACTION GUIDELINES

For trainers with clients who have disability it is often not the ability to adapt the activity that is the problem. Problems normally arise when interacting with individuals with disabilities. Even though the list of disabilities is endless, there are certain ones that trainers might come across that can be grouped together. These areas include wheelchair use, hearing, speech or vision impairment and learning disability and the use of simple guidelines related to each of these areas can be helpful.

Speech impairment

Speech disabilities can have a myriad of different causes. A stroke, for example, may cause a speech disability that others find difficult to understand.

Wheelchair users

One of the main misconceptions surrounding wheelchair use is that only those with mobility problems use wheelchairs. Just pop to your local sports centre and you will see non-disabled people using wheelchairs in a variety of sports. In statistical terms, less than 8% of disabled people are wheelchair users.

The use of wheelchairs in sporting situations can be traced back to the late 1940s when a German Neurologist, the late Sir Ludwig Guttmann, introduced sport as part of the reha-

Speech impairment: interaction guidelines

- Be patient when communicating.
- Don't speak for the client. Allow them to answer in their own time.
- Short questions (or closed questions as they are known) that require short answers or a nod or shake of the head are recommended.
- Never pretend to understand if you do not. Just be honest.

Wheelchair users: interaction guidelines

- Any equipment a client may use, such as a wheelchair, is part of their personal space.
- Don't physically interact with a client's body or equipment unless you're asked to do so or you ask first.
- When speaking to a client in a wheelchair, try to be at their eye level without kneeling.
- If a client transfers out of a wheelchair, to a car, for example, leave the wheelchair within easy reach.
- Remind clients to drink regularly as overheating often occurs.
- Encourage changing seat position often as circulation may be poor.

bilitation of his patients at the National Spinal Injuries Centre at Stoke Mandeville Hospital. In 1948 he organised the first national competition which eventually led to the first Paralympic Games (i.e. games running in parallel) in 1960 which were held in Rome. Guttmann is now

Hearing impairment: interaction guidelines

- To get attention, tap the client on the shoulder or wave your hand in front of them.
- Find out if the client prefers sign language, gesturing, writing or speaking.
- Look directly at the client and speak clearly and slowly.
- Speak in a normal tone of voice.
- Try to talk when background noise is low.
- Face the sun if you are outside and try to have light on your face if you are inside.
- Written notes can often help. Do not talk while writing.
- If you have trouble understanding, just let the client know.

Vision impairment: interaction guidelines

- Always identify yourself and others when meeting a client with vision impairment.
- It helps to tell the client that the conversation is finished and that you are moving.
- When you give help, allow the client to take your arm so you can lead.
- When offering a seat, place the client's hand on the back or arm of the seat.
- Try to be consistent in each session with things like leaving equipment in the same place.
- Use 'clock clues' to help orient in the room.
- Use large print when writing or giving notes.

widely acknowledged as the father of the Paralympics and sport for the disabled.

Hearing impairment

According to the English Federation of Disability Sport there are approximately 9 million deaf and hard of hearing people in the UK. The range of hearing impairment is vast and can range from mild hearing loss to what is considered to be 'profound deafness'. Some individuals who have only a mild degree of hearing loss might rely on the use of hearing aids whereas others might rely on speech reading (lip reading), sign language or a combination of both.

Vision impairment

As with hearing impairment, there is a wide range of vision impairment. Some individuals may only have a limited vision and just require the use of corrective lenses (glasses or contact lenses) whereas other individuals may have a total loss of vision. In the case of total loss of vision, the amount of dependence on others to help with daily activities can vary dramatically between individuals from the use of a cane or stick to guide dogs or carer assistance.

Learning disability

A learning disability is a condition in which the brain does not develop as it should and may occur as a result of brain injuries, infections, trauma, genetic or developmental problems or difficulties with speech and language. Unfortunately, there is often a stigma attached to the term 'learning difficulties' but this is an extremely common condition as it is estimated that there are approximately 1.5 million people in the UK who have a learning disability and about 200 babies are born with a learning disability every year. It is also an area that is rapidly gaining more awareness, which will hopefully help to reduce the negative connotations. According to the English Federation of Disability Sport, about 17% of people with a learning disability are employed and more disturbing is the statistic that about 9 out of 10 people with a learning disability get bullied.

ACTIVITY GUIDELINES

Many individuals with disabilities regularly take part in organised sports or activities. As with anyone, cardiovascular capacity and muscular strength and endurance are components of fitness that should be addressed to help with the particular chosen sport or activity. For example, there are wheelchair variations that are now available for sports such as cycling, distance events, basketball, tennis and even skiing. It is obvious that these are all activities that require specific components of fitness to be developed.

In terms of developing cardiovascular capacity, there are now many health or fitness centres that have machines that are adaptable for this specific purpose. For muscular strength and endurance training, the use of free weights, resistance bands and resistance machines (these can provide support while lifting) are all effective. Although there are many different cardiovascular and resistance exercises that can be done depending on the equipment available, there are some typical exercises for wheelchair users that can be done with equipment commonly found in most fitness centres. Figures 10.3 to 10.5 give an example of just some of the cardiovascular exercises that can be done.

Arm cranking:

There are many types of arm cranking cardio machines in gyms nowadays. The person sits in the seat of the machine and uses their arms to turn the crank (a bit like pedals on a bike).

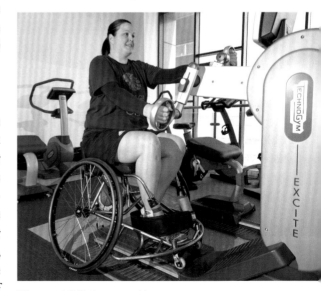

Figure 10.3 Arm cranking

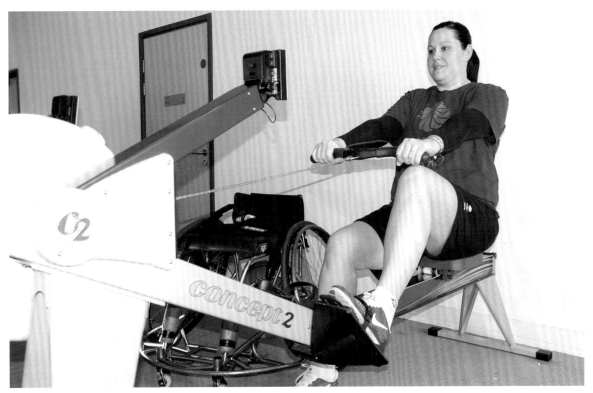

Figure 10.4 Rowing

Rowing/kayaking

Some rowing machines can now be adapted to fix the seat in place. There are also other machines that are kayaking specific.

Distance 'wheeling'

Wheelchairs with 3 wheels are now available to enable the user to do any type of distance event. These wheelchairs make it possible for the person to steer while maintaining the speed.

The range of resistance type exercises that wheelchair users can do with resistance bands or free-weights is endless. With resistance machines, however, this will depend on the availability at the centre of choice. Exercises 10.1 to 10.5 give a description of the more common resistance

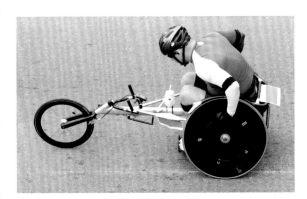

Figure 10.5 Wheeling

exercises that can be done with certain resistance machines (or in this particular case the resistance bands if machines are not available).

Exercise 10.1 Lat pull down

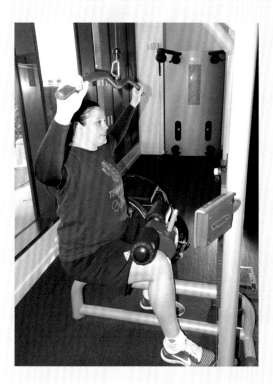

Exercise 10.2 Chest press

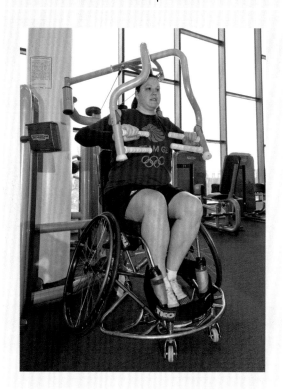

- To work the large muscles of the back, sit at a lat pull down machine and extend the arms to take hold of the bar or a resistance band wrapped around any fixed point.
- Pull the bar or bands down to chin level.
- Extend the arms to the start position controlling the movement all the way.

- To work the large muscles of the chest, sit at a bench or chest press machine and take hold of the handles or resistance band.
- Extend the arms forward until they are at full extension.
- Let the arms return to the start point but control the movement all the way.
- At the start point try and keep the hands within peripheral vision as this will protect the shoulder joint.

Exercise 10.3 Shoulder press

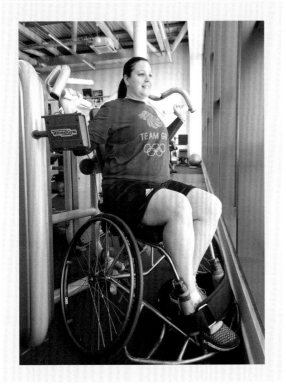

Exercise 10.4 Tricep push

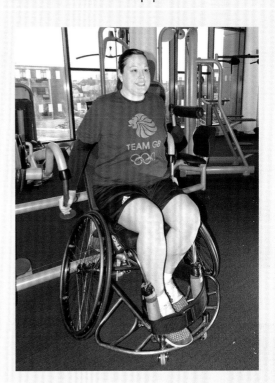

- To work the muscles of the shoulder, sit at a shoulder press machine and take hold of the handles or the resistance band that is passed under the seat.
- Extend the arms above the head.
- Let the arms return to the start point but control the movement all the way.
- For the start point, try and keep the upper arms parallel with the floor.

- To work the muscles at the back of the arms, sit at a tricep push machine and push down on the handles or the resistance band that is anchored overhead.
- Control the arm movement back to the start position.

Exercise 10.5 Bicep curl

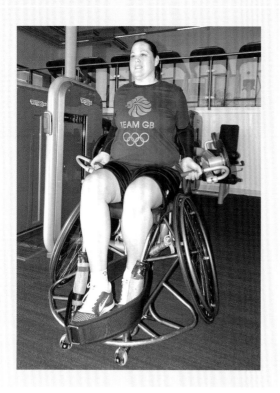

- To work the muscles of the front of the arms sit at a bicep curl machine, take hold of the handles or bands and lift them towards the face.
- Control the arm movement back to the start position.

For those that are not familiar with resistance training, especially with the use of resistance machines, there are a few general guidelines that can be followed:

- Take advice from a qualified trainer when selecting the appropriate weight for each exercise.
- Some makes of machine allow for the seat to be removed so that the wheelchair can be used as the seat.
- If the wheelchair is to be used, make sure that the individual is correctly strapped in.
- For resistance band exercises, make sure that the band is taut at the starting point of each exercise. Bands come in different thicknesses.
- Grip is often a problem for those with certain disabilities. The use of straps or 'action gloves' can be helpful.
- Try to identify muscles that are weak. These usually include latissimus dorsi, erector spinae and trapezius.

FITNESS TESTING

Most standard fitness tests are suitable depending on the particular disability. However, because of the lower body limitations that are often associated with wheelchair users, aerobic capacity is a component of fitness that is commonly tested. There are various methods that have been used over the years but one such test, designed by Franklin in 1990, known as the 'wheelchair fitness test', allows the individual to be tested in their own wheelchair. The test does allow for an estimation of fitness rating and classification, however, it is also useful for setting a baseline for the individual that can be used to track any future improvement.

TEST BOX – Wheelchair fitness test

Equipment needed: Stopwatch, cones, track or measured distance.

- Place cones around a track at 50 metre intervals to help measuring.
- All participants line up on the start line.
- Participants have to wheel around the track as far as they can for 12 minutes.
- Record the distance to the nearest 100 metres.

Use the following table to give a fitness rating and an estimate of VO_2.

Table 10.9	Wheelchair fitness classifications		
Miles	Kilometers	Estimated VO_2 (ml/kg/min)	Fitness rating
<0.63	<1.01	<7.7	poor
0.63–0.86	1.01–1.38	7.7–14.5	below average
0.87–1.35	1.39–2.17	14.6–29.1	fair
1.36–1.59	2.18–2.56	29.2–36.2	good
>1.59	>2.57	>36.2	excellent

USEFUL WEBSITES

BAALPE: www.baalpe.org

British Blind Sport: www.britishblindsport.org.uk

British Deaf Sports Council: www.britishdeafsportscouncil.org.uk

British Paralympic Association: www.paralympics.org.uk

British Wheelchair Sports Foundation (wheel-power): www.wheelpower.org.uk

CP Sport: www.cpsport.org

Disability Sport England: www.disabilitysport.org.uk

Disability Sport Wales: www.disabilitysportwales.org

Disability Sports Northern Ireland: www.dsni.co.uk

Down's Syndrome Association: www.downs-syndrome.org.uk.

English Federation of Disability Sport: www.efds.co.uk

Scottish Disability Sport: www.scottishdisabilitysport.com

UK Sports Association for People with Learning Difficulties: www.uksportsassociation.org

DIGESTIVE SYSTEM AND NUTRIENTS

11

THE NOS LEVEL 3 PERSONAL TRAINER CRITERIA COVERED IN THIS CHAPTER ARE:

- The structure and function of the digestive system
- The nutritional requirements and hydration needs of the physical activity programme and how to explain it to clients
- The role of carbohydrate, fat and protein as fuels for aerobic and anaerobic exercise
- A basic understanding of the function and metabolism of micro and macro nutrients
- The calorific/Kilojoule value of nutrients and awareness of terminology used including:
  - UK dietary reference values (DRV)
  - Recommended daily allowance (RDA)
  - Recommended daily intake (RDI)
  - Glycaemic Index
- The relationship between nutrition, physical activity, body composition and health and how to explain it to clients including:
  - links to disease / disease risk factors
  - cholesterol (desirable levels of HDL, LDL, Total Cholesterol: HDL ratio)
  - types of fat
- Why it is important to collect accurate nutritional information about your clients
- Familiarity with food labelling information and its interpretation

THE DIGESTIVE SYSTEM

The digestive system can be thought of as a long tube that passes through the body from the mouth to the rectum. The main role of the digestive system (with the help of various organs) is to digest and absorb nutrients (see page 164 for macro and micronutrients) from food. Digestion can be described as the mechanical and chemical breakdown of food into smaller components that are more easily absorbed into a blood stream.

THE DIGESTION PROCESS

Although an extremely complex process, ingestion, digestion, assimilation and excretion of food (plus synthesis of certain nutrients such as vitamin B12) can be described in simple terms. As can be seen in figure 11.1 the process of digestion starts in the mouth as salivary glands (along with chewing, known as 'mastication') produce enzymes that break down foods. From the mouth food passes into the stomach where various acids and enzymes are released to further the breakdown process into a thick liquid known as 'chyme'. This partially digested food then passes through the pyloric sphincter (a circular muscular exit) which regulates the amount and speed of chyme leaving the stomach to pass into the duodenum.

It is here that the pancreas and digestive tract release various enzymes designed to breakdown each of the different macronutrients and the gall bladder secretes bile to help break down fats. Once this has taken place the mix of nutrients then passes into the small intestine where final breakdown and much of the absorption of the nutrients takes place (up to 95%). From the small intestine, any remaining food which has not been absorbed moves into the large intestine in which faeces are produced and excreted via the anal sphincter. Movement of food through the digestive system happens mainly as a result of smooth muscle contraction known as 'peristaltic' action. As macronutrients differ in their rate of digestion and absorption, the process of each should be considered separately.

The digestion and absorption of protein

Proteins are made up of differing lengths of amino acid chains and the aim of digestion is to break down the chains into individual amino acids. This process does not occur in the same place but rather follows a progressive breakdown as protein makes its way through the digestive system (as shown in table 11.1).

When amino acid chains are greatest in length (more than 100 amino acids) they are known as 'polypeptides'. When food enters the mouth saliva is secreted which, with the help of chewing helps to physically break down the food into smaller pieces, known as 'bolus'. When a bolus travels to the stomach, hydrochloric acid and

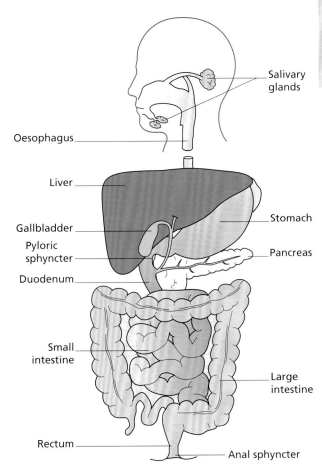

Figure 11.1 The digestion system

Table 11.1	Protein digestion process (simplified)	
Enzyme	**Protein**	**Organ**
Saliva and chewing helps physical breakdown	Polypeptide (>100 amino acids)	Mouth
Hydrochloric acid and Pepsin	Chains become smaller	Stomach
Proteases (group of enzymes mainly trypsin and chymotrypsin)	Peptides (<100 amino acids)	Pancreas
Peptidase (group of enzymes)	Di-peptide (2 amino acids)	Small intestine
	Single amino acid	Circulatory system and liver

pepsin (sometimes referred to as 'gastric juice') are secreted, which acts to start the breakdown of the amino chains. The chime mixture then travels to the duodenum where various enzymes (proteases) are secreted from the pancreas to break down the chains still further. By the time this has passed through the duodenum it has been broken down into chains of only two amino acids (known as dipeptides). The final stage of digestion is performed by the brush border (so called because small projections called villi resemble a brush) of the small intestine. Once in the small intestine, a group of enzymes known as 'peptidases' break down the dipeptides into single amino acids which are small enough to be absorbed into the blood stream. It has been demonstrated that amino acids from natural food sources are absorbed more efficiently than those in supplement form (if numbers are equal). The liver plays an important role as it monitors the levels of absorbed amino acids and adjusts the rate of metabolism to the requirements of the body.

The digestion and absorption of fat

Most of the fats in our diet are made up of triglycerides (see page 164). Triglycerides consist of three fatty acid chains attached to a glycerol backbone. Each fatty acid is attached by what is known as an 'ester bond' (by the process of condensation and hydrolysis). Digestion of fat differs from that of protein in that only one enzyme (lipase) is used to break down the bonds between the fatty acids and the glycerol backbone. As with protein, chewing helps to physically break down the food, however, unlike protein, the enzyme lingual lipase secreted in the mouth starts the initial breakdown of the fat. Once in the stomach, lipase that is trapped inside the food bolus can continue to work which is why chewing is an important process. The emptying of fat from the stomach into the duodenum is controlled (by the pyloric sphincter) as a large amount of fat is more difficult to break down. This is why fat gives the feeling of being full for longer (satiating effect) as it remains in the stomach for longer. In the duodenum lipase is secreted from the pancreas to further breakdown the fat into glycerol and fatty acids. The gall bladder also releases a substance called bile, which coats the fats (forming small droplets called miscelles) to prevent them combining to make large droplets and also helps to trap lipase to act on the fat. This is known as 'emulsification' and is aided by stomach acids (chemical hydrolysis) and mechanical movement. Again, the liver plays an important part as it helps to regulate the level of bile within the gall bladder. The miscelles then travel to the small intestine where they are able to diffuse across the intestinal wall.

Once across the intestinal wall triglycerides are re-formed (along with protein, phospholipids and cholesterol) to be transported in the circulatory system (lacteal and lymphatic). The percentages of the reformed 'packages' differ but are collectively known as 'lipoproteins' as can be seen in figure 11.2. A chylomicron which is made up mainly of triacylglycerol is too big to be transported in the circulatory system so is transported back to the liver (via the terminal lymph system) to be repackaged into a VLDL (very low density lipoprotein) which can move around the body in the circulatory system. Once nutrients in the VLDL have been used it returns to the liver to

Table 11.2	Fat digestion process (simplified)	
Enzymes	**Fat**	**Organ**
Saliva, lingual lipase and chewing helps physical breakdown	Triglyceride (glycerol backbone + 3 fatty acids)	Mouth
Hydrochloric acid and Pepsin	Mixed with lipase now smaller due to chewing action.	Stomach
	Fat release from stomach slowed down to allow smaller quantities to be digested.	Pyloric Sphincter
Pancreatic lipase	Glycerol and fatty acids in duodenum.	Pancreas
Bile	Coats the fat forming small packages called miscelles. Stops fat combining.	Liver and Gall bladder
	Miscelles diffuse across mucosal membrane.	Small intestine
	Fat (triglycerides reformed) and packaged into lipoproteins.	Circulatory system and lymph back to liver

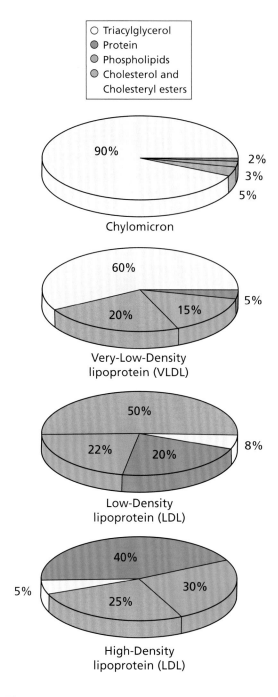

Figure 11.2 Lipoprotein composition (approximate)

Legend:
○ Triacylglycerol
● Protein
◐ Phospholipids
◐ Cholesterol and Cholesteryl esters

Chylomicron: 90%, 2%, 3%, 5%

Very-Low-Density lipoprotein (VLDL): 60%, 5%, 15%, 20%

Low-Density lipoprotein (LDL): 50%, 8%, 20%, 22%

High-Density lipoprotein (LDL): 40%, 30%, 25%, 5%

be repackaged as an LDL, which is then released into the circulation system.

Within this system cholesterol uptake is controlled as HDLs mop up surplus or spare cholesterol and return it to the liver. There are many factors thought to influence the levels of LDLs and HDLs, including genetics, exercise, age, diet, hormone levels and smoking and even though total LDL/HDL levels are important (see pages 168–9) it is the ratio between them that is thought to be more significant.

The digestion and absorption of carbohydrate

The purpose of carbohydrate digestion is to break the carbohydrate (in poly and disaccharide form) down into single sugars known as monosaccharides (see page 169). The process starts in the mouth where enzymes in the saliva (salivary amylase) act on the carbohydrate. Chewing is important as it can increase the carbohydrate breakdown by increasing the surface area to volume ratio of the food and also by trapping saliva in the food bolus that is passed through to the stomach. Once in the stomach the bolus is exposed to hydrochloric acid and pepsin (as with all food) which destroys any amylase that is on the surface of the bolus but not that trapped within. The salivary amylase starts the process of breaking down the polysaccharides into shorter chains which then pass to the duodenum where the pancreas releases pancreatic amylase and the digestive process continues. The chains are further broken down into disaccharides (two sugars combined) which then pass into the small intestine. Once in the small intestine, enzymes known as brush border enzymes break down the disaccharides into monosaccharides (note: there are different enzymes for different disaccharides).

The disacchrides are easily distinguished as their names end in 'ose', for example: maltose, sucrose and lactose, whereas the enzymes that break them down end in 'ase' for example: maltase, sucrase and lactase. The monosaccharides are then absorbed through the small intestine wall where they are transported in the circulatory system back to the liver, which regulates their amount in the blood. Excess monosaccharides can be used for energy production; stored as glycogen in the liver and muscles or converted and stored as fat.

NUTRIENTS

All foods contain chemicals known as nutrients, which are needed for essential processes such as growth and metabolism. Nutrients needed in very small amounts are called micronutrients (vitamins, minerals and fibre) and have no energy content while those that are needed in larger quantities and provide energy are called macronutrients (proteins, fats and carbohydrates). There are many guidelines in relation to the recommended amounts of macronutrients, such as that by the World Health Organisation which suggests an average daily intake (based on the ideal amount of calories) of carbohydrate, fat and protein for the general population should be made up of the following;

- Fats: up to 30% (less than 10% from saturated fats)
- Protein: 10–15%
- Carbohydrate: 55–60% (less than 10% from simple sugars)

Table 11.3	Carbohydrate digestion process (simplified)	
Enzymes	**Carbohydrate**	**Organ**
Salivary amylase and chewing helps physical breakdown	Polysaccharides, disaccharides and monosaccharides do not require much digestion.	Mouth
Hydrochloric acid and Pepsin	Polysaccharides are broken down into shorter chains. Any amylase on the surface broken down by pepsin.	Stomach
Pancreatic amylase	Polysaccharide further broken down and pass into small intestine.	Pancreas
Brush border enzymes maltase, sucrase, lactase	Disaccharides and monosaccharides (single and double sugars).	Small intestine
Diffuse across mucosal membrane	Monosaccharides (glucose, fructose and galactose).	Circulatory system and liver

There are other guidelines, however, such as those by Sharkey and Gaskill 2007, that are slightly different and also give guidelines for daily intake related to performance as can be seen in table 11.4.

All calories should come from macronutrients which should be balanced (as in the plate model, page 182) enough in the diet to provide the necessary amounts of micronutrients as well. Vitamins (listed in table 11.6) are organic substances that are essential in the metabolism of fats, carbohydrates and protein, and have numerous other functions such as blood clotting, protein synthesis and bone formation.

PROTEIN, FAT AND CARBOHYDRATE SOURCES FOR EXERCISE

The three macronutrients (protein, fat and carbohydrate) are all sources of the main energy currency in the body known as adenosine tri-phosphate or ATP (trainers should be familiar with this term). At rest and at lower intensities of aerobic exercise, fat is the predominant fuel source for the production of ATP energy. The cross-over point from predominantly fat as the main fuel source to predominantly carbohydrate can depend on many factors such as the fitness of the individual but typically occurs between 50–70% VO_2 max. At an intensity where carbohydrate becomes the main fuel source it is known as anaerobic exercise. For a client with the goal of trying to reduce body fat, the recommendation therefore would be to choose a suitable mode of aerobic exercise that the individual prefers, for example jogging, cycling or swimming. The choice of intensity would depend on the individual's fitness level, but exercising at an average intensity of around 70% HR max should allow them to exercise for at least 30 minutes (this can be made up of 3 x 10 minute sessions) and, as

Table 11.4	Recommended daily energy intake for typical and performance diets	
Component	Performance diet (% total cals)	Typical diet (% total cals)
Carbohydrate	55–60	45–50
Fat	25–30	35–40
Protein	15	10–15

a result, be effective in inducing fat loss until they are capable of training at higher intensities.

There are often conflicting messages relating to the use of protein as a fuel source. This is possible (in some cases up to 10% of that required) but it should be noted that this only occurs in the absence of carbohydrates (i.e. on low-carbohydrate diets) which in the long term has been shown to result in the wasting away of lean tissue. It should also be mentioned at this point that a lack of carbohydrate in the diet can also result in incomplete fat breakdown which results in an accumulation of ketone bodies which can increase body fluid acidity and create harmful conditions (acidosis). This type of 'ketosis' as it is better known is typical of low-carbohydrate diets.

Protein

The term 'protein' translates from the Greek meaning 'of prime importance'. A protein is made up of chains of individual amino acids, which are small molecules that act as the building blocks of any cell needed for growth and repair (the body is about 20% protein by weight). The human body is constructed of about 20 different amino acids of which there are two different types: essential and non-essential. Non-essential amino acids are amino acids that the body can manufacture, whereas essential amino acids can only be ingested. Protein in our diets comes from both animal sources, such as meat, fish, milk, eggs, and vegetable sources, such as pulses, nuts, seeds and beans, but trainers should be aware that vegetable sources may not contain all essential amino acids.

Protein requirements

Various studies have been carried out on the protein needs of various people yet there is still debate in this area. The Department of Health at the International Conference of Food, Nutrition and Sports Performance suggested the following guidelines:

- 0.75–1 g/kg/day – for those who are sedentary
- 1.2–1.8 g/kg/day – for those who engage in regular endurance activities
- 2.0–2.4 g/kg/day – for those who engage in regular strength and power activities

Dietary issues

A typical UK diet contains between 11 and 14% of energy as protein. Too little protein in the diet has been linked to poor stamina, low energy levels, reduced resistance to infection and the rate of healing decreasing, however, a healthy balanced diet is generally considered to contain enough protein without the need for supplementation. High protein levels are common in those who do supplement but this can lead to stress on the kidneys as a result of the excess production of urine. Trainers should advise clients with high protein intakes to regularly check the colour of their urine. A dark-coloured and pungent urine

indicates a potentially excessive protein intake. The trainer should also inform the client that protein is usually high in fat and excess protein is normally stored as fat.

Fat

The correct term for fat is actually 'lipid', which comes from the Greek 'lipos' meaning fat. Digested fats are transported in the bloodstream as triglycerides and are either stored or burned as fuel. A triglyceride is made up of a glycerol backbone with three fatty acid chains attached. It is the structure of the chain which determines if the fat is saturated or unsaturated (sub-divided into mono and polyunsaturated). Saturated fats are normally solid at room temperature, while unsaturated fats are liquid at room temperature. Vegetable oils are examples of unsaturated fats, while lard and animal fat (as well as palm and coconut oil) are examples of saturated fats. Fat is a very important component of the diet as it has a number of important roles such as:

- an energy source (predominantly in aerobic exercise)
- cell membrane structure
- protection for the nervous system
- production of hormones
- transportation of fat soluble vitamins A, D, E and K
- source of essential fatty acids (these are fats that cannot be synthesised by the body so must be obtained in the diet in sources such as seeds, grains and oily fish).

Fat requirements

The WHO guidelines state that up to 30% (approx 1/3) of our total energy intake should come from fat; however, many sources show that in the UK more than 40% of energy intake in the diet comes from fat. It is useful to be able to calculate these percentages in terms of grams of fat in the diet. The following calculation shows a quick method to calculate an average daily fat intake:

Calculating the average daily fat intake

Example: If a client's energy requirements are 2,400Kcal per day, then the calculation would be as follows:

- **Step 1:** 2,400 divided by 3 (approx ⅓) = 800Kcal
- As 1g fat = 9 Kcal of energy then:
- **Step 2:** 800 divided by 9 = 88.88g of fat per day

The Department of Health (1991a) on the other hand recommends that we consume a maximum of 35% of our calories from fat bearing in mind that the intake in the UK is close to 40%.

Dietary issues

Instructors should be aware that foods containing high fat levels are generally tastier but as fat contains more than twice the number of calories per gram compared to carbohydrate or protein, the risk of obesity is greater. As obesity increases the risk of many conditions such as diabetes, coronary heart disease, high blood pressure and various cancers, it is recommended that fats in the diet are limited, in particular a type known as trans fatty acids. This is a type of fat that has essentially undergone a transformation from its original state, such as from the hydrogenation process used in the manufacture of hard margarines, some biscuits and pastries. There is also a link between high levels of saturated fat and high levels of cholesterol. Cholesterol is a type of lipid found in all of us as it is an essential compound needed for important roles in the body such as making cells (the body's 'building blocks') and hormones, which act as important chemical messengers in the body. Both triglycerides and cholesterol move between the intestine and the liver via the bloodstream. On their own they are not soluble in the blood, therefore, they must combine with protein to form various lipoproteins in order to be transported through the blood. When blood is being tested for cholesterol levels it is really the lipoproteins that are being measured. The main types of lipoproteins that are often measured are known as:

- Very low density lipoprotein (VLDL) which is the main carrier of triglyceride.
- Low-density lipoprotein (LDL) which is the 'bad' carrier of cholesterol.
- High-density lipoprotein (HDL) known as the 'good' carrier of cholesterol.

Specific blood tests need to be carried out (by a qualified person) in order to determine the overall total cholesterol level. As can be seen in table 11.5 it is desirable for an individual to have less than 5.2mmol/l, however, individual levels of LDL-cholesterol and HDL-cholesterol should also be identified as the ratio between them is important. For example, if a person with a borderline high total cholesterol level has a good ratio of LDL to HDL, then it is considered to be healthier than having a borderline high total cholesterol level

Table 11.5	Cholesterol classifications (Units are mmol/l of blood)		
Lipoprotein	**Desirable**	**Border**	**Abnormal**
Total cholesterol	< 5.2	5.2–6.5	> 6.5
LDL cholesterol	< 3.0	3.0–5.0	> 5.0
HDL cholesterol	> 1.0	0.9–1.0	< 0.9

with a poor ratio of LDL to HDL. A ratio of less than 3 to 1 (LDL to HDL) is considered to be good.

High lipid levels in the blood are known to speed up a process called 'atherosclerosis', or hardening of the arteries. Arteries, if undamaged, are normally smooth on the inside, which allows blood to flow easily through them. If the arteries get damaged in any way (smoking can cause damage for example), a substance called 'plaque' can form on the inside walls at the site of the damage. Plaque is just the collective term for substances such as lipids that can 'stick' to the artery walls as they flow through the bloodstream. If plaque continues to build up (as can be seen in figure 11.3), the arteries can narrow and stiffen which in turn can reduce the blood flow and lead to serious consequences such as angina, stroke and heart attack. The instructor should explain in simple terms the effects of cholesterol to clients and also point out that regular exercise has been shown to increase HDL levels (and in some cases reduce LDL levels) thereby reducing the risk of developing atherosclerosis and heart attack.

Carbohydrates

The word 'carbohydrate', or carbs as they are commonly known, reflects the fact that it is made up of carbon and water. When carbs are digested they form saccharides, or sugars as they are usually referred to. Saccharides are then sub-divided into monosaccharides (single sugars) such as glucose, fructose and galactose, which are the only carbohydrates that can be absorbed into the bloodstream, and disaccharides (two sugars) such as lactose, sucrose and maltose that are digestible.

There is another category of carbohydrate known as fibre or non-starch-polysaccharide (NSP) which is indigestible. Fibre moves through the digestive system where it absorbs water and toxins to be excreted from the body. Fibre also helps get rid of cholesterol and fats out of the body (by absorbing them) thus reducing the risk of heart disease.

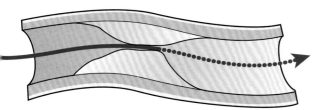

Figure 11.3 An artery wall with plaque build up

When glucose enters the bloodstream it provides energy for the following functions:

- the brain and nervous system (requires 500–600 Kcals daily)
- the liver and digestive system (requires 300–400 Kcals daily)
- muscular contractions (requirement depends upon activity level)

When glucose is stored in the liver and muscles it is called glycogen. The body is capable of storing about 1600kcals of energy as glycogen (about 1200kcals in the muscles and 400kcals in the liver) which is sufficient for the short term only (about 24 hours), which is why carbohydrates are important in the daily diet.

Carbohydrate requirement
The WHO guidelines state that 55–60% (approximately two thirds) of our total energy intake should come from carbohydrate. It is useful to be able to calculate these percentages in terms of grams of carbohydrate in the diet. The following calculation shows a quick method to calculate an average daily carbohydrate intake.

Calculating the average daily carbohydrate intake
Example: If a client's energy requirements are 2,400Kcal per day, then the calculation would be as follows:

- **Step 1:** 55–60% of 2,400 = 1320–1440Kcal
- As 1 gram of carbohydrate = 4Kcal of energy then
- **Step 2:** 1320–1440 divided by 9 = 330–360g of carbohydrate per day

More active people require a higher level of carbohydrate than others to replenish the glycogen that is used during exercise. Clients who exercise for long periods of time should be encouraged to consume carbs during exercise in order to avoid fatigue.

Dietary issues
Carbohydrates that are digested quickly are usually referred to as 'simple carbohydrates' (such as refined foods like cakes, soft drinks and sweets) and those that are digested slowly are referred to as 'complex carbohydrates' (such as grains, pasta, cereals, etc). Simple sugars require little digestion, and when eaten the glucose level in the blood rises rapidly. In response, the pancreas secretes a large amount of insulin to keep blood glucose levels from rising too high. This large insulin response in turn tends to make the blood sugar fall to levels that are too low leading to an adrenalin surge, which in turn can cause nervousness and irritability. Prolonged eating behaviour such as this is strongly linked to Type II diabetes, as is obesity, therefore, clients should be made aware of this. Also let them know that research has shown that regular exercise can help to reduce the onset of diabetes by regulating blood sugar and obesity levels.

Glycaemic index
Essentially the Glycaemic Index (GI) is a ranking of foods from 0–100, based on the rate at which a carbohydrate is broken down. Glucose has a GI of 100 and all carbohydrate foods are compared to this. A food which has a glycaemic index of 85 or over is regarded as high GI; moderate GI is 60–84 and low GI is less than 60. Foods that have a high GI are absorbed into the bloodstream quickly and therefore affect the insulin response mentioned earlier. Foods that are low GI are absorbed at a

slower rate and do not affect the insulin response as much. It is widely recommended to select foods that are low in GI as often as possible (visit www.glycemicindex.com). Instructors should encourage clients to use the GI when making food choices. Low GI diets are recommended for diabetic subjects and they inhibit the sense of hunger after eating and increase endurance during exercise. The use of low GI foods is encouraged as it has been shown to reduce the elevation of insulin and lipids after a meal, but all GI foods (with an emphasis on low-moderate) should be consumed in a balanced diet, as foods with a high GI value have a role in replenishing muscle glycogen quickly during or after exercise.

Vitamins

Vitamins are organic substances that are normally categorised into two groups based on how they are absorbed and used by the body: fat-soluble such

Table 11.6	Potential problems related to vitamin deficiency	
Vitamin	**Main use**	**Deficiency**
Vitamin A (fat soluble)	Retinol: found in plants such as carrots. Essential for vision in dim light and is also required for skin, mucus membranes and growth	Night blindness (xerophthalmia)
Vitamin B (water soluble)	B1: Thiamine: release of energy from carbohydrates, especially important for the brain and nerve function	Beriberi (nervous system disorder)
	B2: Riboflavin: release of energy, especially from protein and fat	Problems with lips, tongue, skin
	B3: Niacin: energy release from nutrients	Pellagra (skin disorder)
	B5: Pantothenic acid: utilised in metabolic pathways	Fatigue
	B6: Pyridoxine: used in many biological reactions is especially associated with amino acid metabolism	Skin problems
	B7: Biotin: cell growth and fat metabolism	Hair loss, dermatitis
	B9: Folic Acid: important for protecting the new foetus	Diarrhoea, anaemia
	B12: Cyanocobalamin: important for folate metabolism	Pernicious anaemia
Vitamin C (water soluble)	Ascorbic acid: immune system, aids wound healing and iron absorption	Scurvy (sickness and skin disorders)
Vitamin D (fat soluble)	Calciferol: Promotes calcium absorption from food.	Rickets (bone softening)
Vitamin E (fat soluble)	Tocopherol: protective effect for cell membranes.	Malabsorption of fats, anaemia.
Vitamin K (fat soluble)	Menaquinone: especially required to produce blood clotting proteins.	Poor blood clotting, internal bleeding.

as A, D, E and K and water-soluble such as B and C. The main difference is that water-soluble vitamins can't be stored, therefore, the body keeps what it needs and excretes the surplus whereas fat-soluble vitamins can be stored for future use. In the case of research, deficiencies have been linked to many problems such as those shown in table 11.6. Healthy balanced diets are considered to be adequate (in terms of vitamin intake) for most people; however, it is sometimes recommended that certain people who may be deficient take supplements in order to get their recommended daily allowance. The instructor should be aware that in large doses, some vitamins have known side-effects, however, the likelihood of consuming too much of any vitamin from food is remote and not common. Supplementation can cause an excess of certain vitamins which is potentially harmful and the body requires large amounts of energy to excrete these.

Minerals

There are a number of minerals (inorganic elements) derived from the digestion of certain

Table 11.7	Mineral and their functions
Mineral	**Common function**
Calcium	Used by teeth, bones. Muscle and nerve activity. Blood clotting.
Chloride	Metabolism (the process of turning food into energy).
Copper	Oxygen transportation.
Fluorine	Strengthens teeth.
Iron	Transports oxygen in red blood cells. Protein metabolism.
Iodine	Thyroid function, Metabolism, growth and energy production.
Magnesium	Used in enzyme activity and muscle function. Protein building.
Manganese	Has a role in the body's anti-oxidant defences.
Molybdenum	Involved in the metabolism of DNA.
Phosphorus	Present in bones and teeth, a component of all cells.
Potassium	Important for brain and nerve function.
Selenium	Anti-oxidant, growth and metabolism, pancreas function.
Sodium	Regulation of body water content and nerve function.
Zinc	Growth and repair, taste perception, anti-oxidant, foetal development.

foods that our bodies must have in order to carry out a range of functions. Table 11.7 lists and describes the common functions associated with specific minerals. Minerals are often lacking in the diet, which leads to various problems such as osteoporosis – lack of calcium – and anaemia – lack of iron intake. Other minerals such as sodium tend to be over-consumed by the majority of the population, which is a concern as high sodium intake has been linked to hypertension.

Water

Water is considered to be the sixth and most important nutrient as it is important in sustaining life and makes up between 40–70% of the total body mass depending on age, gender and body composition. Many metabolic processes in the body require water to be present, especially digestion and absorption of nutrients and this can be affected if the body becomes too dehydrated (from the Greek word 'hydro' meaning water). Effects of dehydration can include:

- Decreased ability to sweat
- Reduced blood flow to kidneys
- Decrease in muscle glycogen
- Increased risk of heat stroke
- Impaired cardiac function

As water is lost through processes such as urination, exhalation and evaporation through the skin, etc., it must be replaced every day in the form of food (many foods contain water, especially fruits) and fluids. The plate model (see page 181) does show some fluids, such as milk and fruit juice, however, water, tea and coffee are major contributors to fluid intake (not alcohol, as it is a diuretic, which means it promotes dehydration). Even though there is no exact recommendation about the amount of total fluid that should be drunk in a day, general guidelines often refer to 6–8 glasses, cups or mugs of fluid. Instructors should be aware, however, that many food sources such as fruit and vegetables contain high amounts of water, therefore, an individual with high daily intakes would probably need less fluid in the form of drinks. In light of the lack of clear guidelines it is the intention of the National Institute of Clinical Health and Excellence to publish its first hydration guidelines in 2013.

Dehydration

Symptoms of dehydration are often difficult to identify, however, typical symptoms of mild dehydration include headaches, decreased blood pressure (hypotension), dark or decreased urine volume, tiredness and dizziness. In cases of moderate dehydration, urine output can cease and fainting can occur. As dehydration becomes increasingly severe, the heart rate can speed up to compensate for the decrease in blood pressure and nausea and delirium could begin as shown in table 11.8. There are also serious recorded effects of long-term dehydration. According to the National Confidential Enquiry into Patient Outcomes and Death (2009) severe dehydration is a leading contributory factor in acute kidney injury that can lead to permanent kidney damage and even death, as evidenced by the deaths of 816 hospital patients in England and Wales in 2009 (specific details of cause of death not given). There is a simple method of checking the amount of fluid lost as a result of an exercise session (equating to percentage of body weight loss) by checking body weight immediately before and after exercise.

Figure 11.4 is an example of a typical recording sheet (for a blank template please visist: www.bloomsbury.com/9781408187234) that can be used but it is important to try and record as much information relevant to the session as possible for future reference. For example, it is important to know the temperature of the environment, as this can influence the rate at which fluid is lost

Table 11.8	Typical effects of dehydration related to % body mass loss
% loss	**Typical effects**
1	Thirst, increased heat regulation, decline in endurance performance.
2	Increased heat regulation, increased thirst, decreased endurance performance and co-ordination.
3	Further increase in the above.
4	Exercise performance decreases by up to 20 – 30% (includes muscular strength).
5	Headaches, nausea, fatigue.
6	Weakness, loss of thermoregulation, vomiting.
7+	Possible collapse.

SESSION FLUID LOSS RECORDING SHEET

Client name   Date

Environment: Gym Temp: 18.5°C   Type of session: Cardio Fluid intake: 750ml

Step 1   Pre-session weight in lbs = 180lbs

Step 2   Post-session weight in lbs = 175lbs

Step 3   Weight lost: Pre-weight (step 1) minus post-weight (step 2) = 5lbs

Step 4   % body weight lost = weight lost (step 3) ÷ pre-weight (step 1) x 100 = 2.77%

Step 5   Millilitres fluid lost: weight lost (step 3) x 452 = 2260ml

% loss (step 4) = 2.77% Fluid loss (step 5) = 2260ml

Figure 11.4 Session fluid loss record sheet

through sweating. In the example, the client's starting weight prior to the exercise session was 180lbs. Following the session it can be seen that the client showed a 5lb loss as their post measurement weight was 175lb. Dividing the weight lost (5lbs) by the pre-session weight (180lbs) and multiplying by 100 gives a total percentage loss of 2.77% (can round up to 2.8%). This can also be calculated in millilitres (ml) of fluid which in this case equates to a loss of 2262ml (see fluid loss record sheet for calculation). As the intake of fluid during the session was only 750ml (as recorded on the sheet) it would make sense to encourage the client to maintain fluid intake after the session had finished in order to make up the deficit. It would also make sense to advise the client to drink more during future sessions to minimise the net fluid loss because, as can be seen in table 11.8, a fluid loss approaching 3% can affect performance.

Fluid loss during endurance-type sessions usually exceeds fluid intake, therefore, it is recommended to try and minimise the net loss. It is unlikely that the client will take in more than they lose as it will be extremely difficult to drink such amounts.

As exercise can cause a greater loss of water than when at rest, steps must be taken to ensure clients are adequately hydrated not just during exercise sessions but before and afterwards. Due to the lack of clear definitive guidelines (and the forthcoming NICE guidelines), the majority of research would suggest following simple steps to help to prevent dehydration:

- Do not rely on thirst as an indicator that a drink is needed as it is not a reliable method of detecting dehydration.
- Avoid wearing many layers of clothing during exercise as this can cause greater fluid losses. If possible, wear breathable exercise clothing and NO sweat suits.
- Cut down on the intake of drinks such as tea/coffee/alcohol as they are all diuretics which cause the body to lose water.
- Check the colour of urine on a regular basis even though it is only a rough guide. It should be pale in colour rather than a dark yellow/orange, which indicates possible dehydration.
- When undertaking an exercise session try to drink the following:
    - 400–600ml 15 mins prior to the session
    - 100–200 every 15 mins during the session
    - Regular sips in the hour after the session
    - 600–1000ml for every 0.5kg (1.1lb) weight loss
- For exercise sessions of less than 60 mins, water is recommended.
- For exercise sessions of more than 60 mins, sports drinks that contain 6–8% glucose polymer solution and electrolytes have been shown to be useful.

There has been much interest in the use of milk as an effective post-exercise rehydration drink and studies show that it can be more effective that water (Shirreffs et al 2007). This could be useful as studies also show that milk is effective post-exercise drink for protein synthesis (Roy 2008). As with all topics it is advised that trainers regularly access the most up-to-date research recommendations in this particular area.

GUIDELINE NUTRIENT AMOUNTS

Assessing the diet for the correct intake of nutrients can be a complex task and should be done by a qualified person, such as a registered dietician.

However, trainers should be aware of terminology related to nutrient intake such as Dietary Reference Values (DRVs) which is a term that has replaced Recommended Daily Allowances (RDA). In simple terms it is an estimate of the amount of energy and nutrients needed by 'healthy' people in the UK (DoH 1991a). For this report the government undertook a survey to establish the nutrient requirements of the UK population and used three classifications to identify certain levels: Reference Nutrient Intake (RNI), Estimated Average Requirement (EAR) and Lower Reference Nutrient Intake (LRNI) as shown in figure 11.5. Guidelines for DRV's can be found in Report 41: Dietary reference values for food energy and nutrients for the United Kingdom. London HMSO:

- EAR – Estimated Average Requirement. The population survey would show a bell-shaped graph or normal spread of distribution similar to that in figure 11.5. This shows that most people fit in the middle of the graph, which indicates an average level of nutrients would be fine for about 50% of the population.

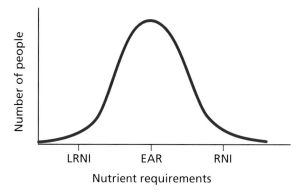

Figure 11.5 The distribution of nutrient requirements within the UK population

- RNI – Reference Nutrient Intake. Because the EAR would only be sufficient for 50% of the population there is a higher nutrient level which would encompass 97.5% of the population and is called the 'reference nutrient intake' or RNI as can be seen in figure 11.5.
- LRNI – Lower Reference Nutrient Intake – There is also the 'lower reference nutrient intake' or LRNI. This level of intake would only be sufficient for 2.5% of the population. If an individual was found to be at this level, it would be a cause for concern as the likelihood of this individual falling into the lower 2.5% of the population who only needed this level of intake would be quite small.

FOOD LABELS

One of the most difficult things for clients (and trainers) is making sense of the myriad of marketing messages on food, which is often conflicting and confusing. Foods in the UK tend to have a lot of information on them, and some of the information can be quite misleading. As the UK is part of the European Union (EU), the laws regarding food labelling are based on EU community legislation, which often undergoes change. Specific information (e.g. name of food, weight or volume, ingredients, date and storage conditions, preparation instructions, name and address of manufacturer, packer or seller, lot number) must appear on food labels by law, although there are some exceptions – in the UK, foods sold loose are currently exempt from many of the food labelling laws (however, some chose to provide this information). Further information can be added optionally, such as the amounts of specific nutrients often as a percentage of the Dietary Reference Value. Some foods also provide information about guideline daily amounts (GDAs). GDAs are derived from the Estimated Average Requirements for energy for men and women aged between 19–50, of normal weight and fitness (2500kcal and 2000kcal respectively). GDAs are intended as guidance to help consumers in their understanding of their recommended daily consumption of energy (calories). For more information visit www.foodstandards.gov.uk.

Sometimes the optional information can be the most misleading, such as in the case of portions of '5-a-day' labels. This particular government campaign was launched to encourage the population to eat a minimum of 5 portions of fruit and/or vegetables every day and as such the Department of Health subsequently developed a specific 5-a-day label with regulations for its use. As there is no law governing this particular labelling, it is often the case that manufacturers are using their own versions of 5-a-day labels to market processed foods that are high in salt, fat and sugar even though they do contain a proportion of the guideline 5-a-day.

Signposting

The Food Standards Agency (FSA) has developed a system for front-of-pack labelling that provides simple visual information on labels about the nutritional content of foods. This is called the traffic light scheme which uses a logo of traffic light colours to indicate low, medium and high amounts of fat (of which saturated), sugar and salt as shown in figure 11.6 which help consumers to make healthier choices.

For instance, a red light on the front of the pack would indicate a high amount of something we should be trying to cut down on. An amber light would indicate the food isn't high or low in

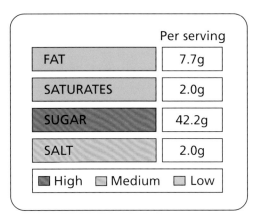

Figure 11.6 Traffic light signposting label

the nutrient (i.e. it's OK some of the time) and a green light means the food is low in that nutrient and is, therefore, the healthier choice. There are conditions however, set out by the FSA that manufacturers are expected to adhere to. For example, the logo must include the following:

- Separate information on fat, saturated fat, sugars and salt
- Red, amber and green colour coding to provide a level information of individual nutrients
- Additional information on the levels of nutrients in a portion of the product

The FSA provides information on the food and drink levels relating to low, medium and high levels as can be seen in table 11.9 which has been adapted from the Food Standards Agency. Front of pack traffic light signpost labelling (technical guidance, Issue 2, 2007).

Label terminology

One of the most confusing things in the food industry is the use of words such as 'low' and

Table 11.9 Food levels per 100g

FOOD	Green (low) grams/100	Amber (medium) grams/100	Red (high) grams/100	Red (high) Per portion
Fat	≤ 3.0	> 3.0 to ≤ 20.0	> 20.0	> 21.0
Saturates	≤ 1.5	> 1.5 to ≤ 5.0	> 5.0	> 6.0
Sugars	≤ 5.0	> 5.0 to ≤ 12.5	> 12.5	> 15.0
Salts	≤ 0.3	> 0.3 to ≤ 1.5	> 1.5	> 2.4
DRINKS	**Green (low) grams/100ml**	**Amber (medium) grams/100ml**	**Red (high) grams/100ml**	
Fat	≤ 1.5	> 1.5 to ≤ 10.0	> 10.0	
Saturates	≤ 0.75	> 0.75 to ≤ 2.5	> 2.5	
Sugars	≤ 2.5	> 2.5 to ≤ 6.3	> 6.3	
Salts	≤ 0.3	> 0.3 to ≤ 1.5	> 1.5	

'fat-free'. This often misleads the public as there is a general conception that anything that has the word low attached to it is regarded as healthy whereas this is not always the case. Trainers should familiarise with the following terms and try to educate clients as to the meanings.

- **Fat-free:** Total fat content per 100g must not exceed 0.15g.
- **Low fat:** Total fat content per 100g (and a normal serving) lower than 5g.
- **Low cal:** Must contain no more than 40kcal per 100g and for drinks no more than 10kcal per 100ml.
- **Reduced fat:** Must contain less than 75% of the fat content of the normal food.

HEALTHY EATING

12

THE NOS LEVEL 3 PERSONAL TRAINER CRITERIA COVERED IN THIS CHAPTER ARE:

- The meaning of key terms including diet, healthy eating, nutrition, balanced diet
- Professional role boundaries with regard to offering nutritional advice to clients
- The basic nutritional principles, key messages and national guidelines that underpin a healthy diet
- An understanding of the National Food Guide
- The main food groups, nutrients they contribute to the diet and portion sizes in the context of the National Food Model
- Practical issues and other factors that influence clients' eating habits and the constraints that may prevent them from achieving their nutritional needs and goals
- Groups of clients at risk of nutritional deficiencies, including:
  - those on severely energy restricted diets
  - those who exclude animal products from their diets
  - those who exclude other food groups from their diet
  - those who are pregnant or lactating
  - older people
  - children
  - those with certain diagnosed medical conditions/diseases
- How to access reliable sources of nutritional information and interpret available information including the distinction between evidence based knowledge versus unsubstantiated anecdote and the marketing claims of suppliers
- The components of energy expenditure and the energy balance equation
- How to determine Basal Metabolic Rate (BMR)
- How to determine energy requirements based on physical activity levels and other relevant factors
- Energy needs/expenditure for different physical activities

- The potential health and performance implications of severe energy restriction, weight loss and weight gain
- A basic awareness of cultural and religious dietary practices
- The importance of communicating the health risks associated with current weight-loss fads and popular diets to clients
- Why detailed or complex dietary analysis that incorporates major dietary change should always be referred to a Registered Dietician
- The circumstances in which you should refer a client on to a GP or an Accredited Sports Dietician and the process you should follow
- Safety, effectiveness and contraindications relating to protein/vitamin supplementation
- Issues that may be sensitive (e.g. yo-yo dieting; eating disorders)
- How to recognise the signs and symptoms of disordered eating and awareness of healthy eating patterns
- Familiarity with the industry guidance note on 'Managing users with suspected eating disorders'.

HEALTHY EATING

In terms of goal setting, many instructors give advice or set specific goals relating to nutrition or dietary habits. The term 'diet' simply relates to what a person eats every day, whereas the term 'nutrition' refers to the provision of certain foods (nutrients) to support life. It should be stressed that the amount of information given to clients should be limited to key areas that follow current government guidelines. For information or advice beyond these key messages instructors should refer clients to qualified people such as registered dieticians, who are qualified to give evidence-based dietary advice, and clinical nutritionists who specialise in the role of nutrition in chronic disease.

One of the main sources of information relating to healthy eating is that of the government Balance of Good Health from the Food Standards Agency (See http://www.food.gov.uk/multimedia/pdfs/bghbooklet.pdf), otherwise known as the 'plate model' as shown in figure 12.1. Dietary goals should always be limited to the advice contained within this model.

THE PLATE MODEL

The government have produced a simple visual way of educating the public about a healthy diet known as the 'plate model'.

The plate model concentrates on five commonly accepted food groups (rather than individual nutrients) and the proportions of these foods that should be eaten from each group:

- Bread, other cereals and potatoes: for example, bread, cereals, potatoes, rice, noodles, pasta.
- Fruit and vegetables: for example, apple, banana, grapes, kiwi, cabbage, peppers, sweet corn, peas.
- Milk and dairy foods: for example, milk, cheese and yoghurt.

- Meat, fish and alternatives: for example, chicken, beef, cod, prawns, eggs, chick peas, nuts.
- Foods containing fat and foods containing sugar: for example, biscuits, jam, margarine, mayonnaise, confectionery, crisps

The intended message is that people should choose a variety of foods from the four largest groups every day (known more commonly as a balanced diet). More foods should be eaten from the bread, other cereals and potatoes group and the fruit and vegetables group compared with the milk and dairy foods group and the meat, fish and alternatives group. Foods in the smallest group (foods containing fat and containing sugar) should be eaten sparingly if they are eaten every day or not eaten too often. It is not necessary to achieve this balance at each meal but it should be applied to food eaten over a day or even a week. Even though public health professionals encourage everyone to eat at least five portions of fruit and vegetables per day (one 'portion' is 80 grams, or a handful) amounts above this can vary depending on energy needs, which are based on age, sex and physical activity levels. As a guide the Food Standards Agency (FSA) (www.foodstandards.gov.uk) has produced a book called *Portion Sizes* in order to help people estimate correct proportion sizes of food in the UK diet.

FACTORS AFFECTING EATING BEHAVIOUR

Trainers must take into account physiological, psychological, social, cultural and sensory factors when dealing with a client's nutritional needs. Trying to change eating behaviour that has been established for many years is extremely difficult and so trainers are advised to study this particular topic in more detail. Nutritional goals may not be achieved if relevant strategies are not implemented in order to address certain factors.

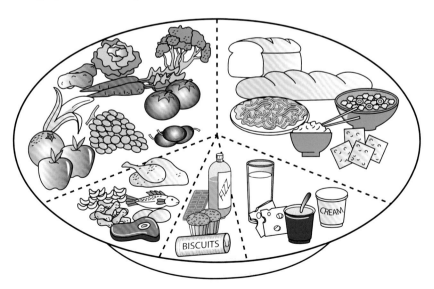

Figure 12.1 The balance of good health plate model

PHYSIOLOGICAL

At a neurological level, the appetite centre in the brain makes a decision as to whether we are hungry or not. Although this system is complex in nature, it is not particularly quick to respond to food being absorbed and can take up to twenty minutes to signal to the brain that the stomach is full. As a result of this it has become very easy to overeat. Eating slowly to allow the signal that we are 'full' to reach the brain is good advice for clients.

PSYCHOLOGICAL

There is a great deal of research which suggests that specific emotions, such as boredom, illness or comfort, is associated with eating behaviour and often links back to childhood. Strategies should be employed that break the link but this is beyond the scope of the trainer.

SOCIAL

The temptation to eat larger portions can be greater when dining out as there is little control over what ingredients are used so try to encourage your client to entertain at home where the number of courses can be restricted and the use of ingredients can be controlled. Trainers should always encourage clients to lead by example rather than follow the choices of others.

CULTURAL

Where we are brought up has a major influence on eating behaviour from a cultural and religious perspective and can affect not only what we eat but how much we eat as well. For example, Christians tend to eat and drink to excess during festivals such as Christmas and Easter. Judaism forbids the eating of pork and foods must be Kosher (prepared under Jewish regulations) before they can be consumed.

Tip

When seeking advice on nutritional issues rely on materials that have been published either in peer-reviewed journals or by government agencies as marketing claims are often exaggerated and not supported by scientific research. Main sources include the Food Standards Agency (www.foodstandards.gov.uk) the National Institute for Health and Clinical Excellence (www.nice.org.uk) and the Department of Health (www.dh.gov.uk).

Hinduism forbids the taking of life for food and therefore, follows a vegetarian diet. Muslims only eat the flesh of ruminant animals (those that digest plant-based foods), excluding pork and also fast for four weeks of every year for a period known as Ramadan when they only eat during the hours of darkness. Trainers should make themselves aware of dietary practices of their clients in relation to cultural or religious preferences.

SENSORY

All senses can affect eating behaviour, which is why marketing is a very powerful tool. Trainers could try to identify which senses clients react most to and remove the source of temptation. Quite often it is just the sight of tempting snacks that is too much for the client, therefore, try to establish where they are coming into contact with the images (magazines, TV, home, shopping, cafes, etc.) and devise strategies to limit the exposure.

NUTRITIONAL DEFICIENCIES

There are many people who may be at risk of nutritional deficiencies for one reason or another.

Table 12.1	Common groups at risk of nutritional deficiencies and associated problems
Group at risk	**Typical associated problem**
Those on severely energy restricted diets such as drastic weight loss or athletes.	As well as missing many essential vitamins and minerals, low-carbohydrate diets also cause toxic effects in the body as a result of ketoacidosis.
Those who exclude animal products from their diets such as vegetarians and vegans.	There are no reported health problems associated with those who follow a diet that includes all essential amino acids and essential fats, however, it is often not easy to do so, therefore, trainers should seek dietary analysis advice. Supplementation of vitamin B12, vitamin D, iron and calcium is often advised.
Those who exclude other food groups from their diet (such as dairy, eggs, fish, poultry).	There are many people who, for a variety of personal cultural or religious reasons, choose to exclude food groups. This can be assessed through the use of food diaries and any strategy decided on an individual basis.
Those who are pregnant or lactating.	Even though exercise can help to reduce the risk of gestational diabetes, do not set weight loss goals during pregnancy (on average add an extra 300Kcals/day). Constipation is common so advise fibre rich foods. Avoid high-sodium foods that increase water retention. No alcohol, caffeine, liver, soft cheese, pâté, raw eggs, certain fish.
Older people.	One of the main concerns is that of osteoporosis. Ensure there is enough calcium and vitamin D for bone strength and carbohydrate to support the exercise required.
Children	Children are often not in control of their own diets and commonly do not achieve a healthy balanced diet (often lacks fruit and veg) which can lead to many associated problems. Trainers should encourage parents to seek nutritional advice when undertaking any programme of exercise if they feel the child's diet is not in line with the plate model.
Those with certain diagnosed medical conditions/diseases	There are many conditions that can occur as a result of deficiencies such as osteoporosis, nervous system disorders, skin disorders, hair loss, diarrhoea, anaemia, blood-clotting problems, etc. Medical advice should always be sought in such cases.

Even though trainers may need to seek professional help with a dietician, it is useful to be aware of the main groups at risk of nutritional deficiencies. Table 12.1 identifies common groups at risk and the typical problems related to those groups.

DIETING DANGERS

Many people use the word 'diet' to mean some type of calorific restriction in order to lose weight. This is the definition that we will use in this section.

For decades common fad diets have become popular based on their marketing claims, however, research often shows that prolonged fasting and diet programmes that severely restrict caloric

Table 12.2 Common fad diets and associated problems	
Marketing claim	**Associated problems**
LOW CARB DIETS (i.e. The Atkins Diet or Ketogenic diets)	
Claims that fat will be used more readily if no carbs are available and that appetite is suppressed due to ketones.	Fat content in the diet is often high leading to increased lipid levels and high calorific content. Acidosis often occurs due to ketones leading to kidney problems. Loss of lean tissue due to protein used as main fuel. Ketogenic diets as they are known are used to treat conditions such as epilepsy but require strict medical supervision.
FOOD COMBINING DIETS	
Suggests is better not to mix carbs and protein in the same meal as enzymes work better in isolation.	Little scientific evidence to support claims. Not feasible to maintain for long periods.
SEVERE LOW-CALORIE DIETS	
Based on the theory that severe calorie restriction will help to break dietary habits and promote quick weight loss.	Weight loss can be severe and nutrient intake depleted leading to many medical problems. Lean tissue loss also common.
HIGH-FIBRE DIETS	
Based on the concept of fibre expanding and creating a feeling of being full thus reducing appetite.	Although fibre in the diet has many benefits, high intakes can reduce mineral absorption and cause bowel discomfort. High water intake needed to help passage through the colon.
FOOD-FOCUSED DIETS (i.e. grapefruit, cabbage soup, etc.)	
Claims that certain foods can increase fat metabolism and are low in calorific content.	Severe lack of many essential nutrients as well as many side other effects such as fainting which can all occur quickly into the diet.

intake can be dangerous as they often result in the loss of large amounts of water, electrolytes, minerals, glycogen stores and other fat-free tissue (including proteins within fat-free tissue) with minimal amounts of fat loss. They can also have the effect of reducing resting metabolic rate leading to a reduction in lean-mass tissue. Even though there are many types of diet circulating at any given time, the trainer should be familiar with some of them and their associated problems as they are often variations of the same theme. Table 12.2 describes some of the more common ones that trainers may be familiar with.

It is important that the trainer educate the client about the health dangers of following a so-called 'diet' and that those who tend to diet in cycles (known as yo-yo dieting) gain weight at quicker rates as resting metabolic rate can be suppressed in order to conserve energy. It is often better to emphasise positive messages as well as educate about the negative aspect. For instance, the following key messages adapted from the ACSM could be used:

- A mild calorie restriction (500–1000kcal) less than the usual daily intake results in a smaller loss of water, electrolytes, minerals and other fat-free tissue, and is less likely to cause medical problems.
- It is recommended that a dual approach be adopted: increase caloric expenditure and decrease caloric intake (but no less than 1200kcal/day).
- Aim for a maximum weight loss 1kg/week (this works out at 8 stone a year!).

EATING DISORDERS
It is possible that instructors may at some time have to deal with the sensitive issue of eating

disorders. Treat any client that comes to you with this issue with tact, sensitivity and, of course, assure him or her that anything they tell you will remain confidential.

Common eating disorders include anorexia nervosa and bulimia nervosa, which are linked closely to obsessive exercise behaviour. Anorexia nervosa (AN) is a condition that usually develops during adolescence and early adulthood and can be described as an eating disorder which is characterised by food restriction (extreme dieting) and a fear of gaining weight. In psychological terms, there is often a distorted body self-perception. Bulimia nervosa (BN) on the other hand is an eating disorder characterised by binge eating and purging (often by vomiting or the use of laxatives). As these conditions require knowledge beyond what is expected from a trainer it is advised to refer this type of client to qualified practitioners. Trainers should, however, be able to identify the characteristics and potential effects of the conditions (as in table 12.3) so that appropriate referral can take place.

The majority of those with AN are younger females although some males do have the condition (about 1 in 20 cases); there are more males with BN but the majority are still females. One of the main differences is that those with AN tend to deny they have the condition whereas those with BN often acknowledge the condition, which makes it easier to deal with.

Diagnosis of the condition is not the responsibility of the trainer. However, the effects of the conditions can be serious, therefore, any concerns must be dealt with as the Code of Ethical Practice states that trainers have a responsibility to ensure as far as possible the safety of the clients with whom they work. Caution must always be used but if a trainer feels that there

Table 12.3	Characteristics and potential effects of anorexia nervosa and bulimia nervosa

Characteristics	Potential effects

ANOREXIA NERVOSA

Physical:
- Extreme weight loss
- Growth retardation
- Delay in puberty
- Facial and body hair
- Amenorrhoea (menstrual irregularities)
- Constantly restless

Psychological:
- Fear of weight gain
- Denial of condition
- Low self-esteem and self-worth
- Depression
- Anxiety
- Distorted body image (think they are bigger)
- Approval seeking

Behavioural:
- Obsessive behaviour (i.e. exercise, calorie counting)
- Perfectionist behaviour
- Social withdrawal
- Poor appetite

Potential effects:
- Reduced performance (in terms of aerobic/ anaerobic and strength).
- Increased risk of infection due to compromised immune system.
- Greater risk of osteoporosis due to decrease in bone density.
- Dehydration (lack of water content in foods).
- Electrolyte (i.e. sodium and potassium) imbalance which can lead to conditions such as cardiac arrhythmias (irregular heart beat) and hypotension (low blood pressure).
- A continued lack of nutrients can also lead to effects such as gastro-intestinal problems, thin brittle hair, and itchy skin.
- Reduced basal metabolic rate.
- Hepatic steatosis – fatty infiltration of the liver.

BULIMIA NERVOSA

Physical:
- Food bingeing followed by vomiting
- Laxative abuse
- Visible tooth decay
- Facial swelling
- Regular weight fluctuations

Psychological:
- Guilt after food bingeing
- Low self-esteem and self-worth
- Depression and often angry
- Distorted body image (think they are bigger)
- Approval seeking

Behavioural:
- Impulsive
- Obsessive exercise behaviour
- Frequent weighing

Potential effects:
- Amenorrhoea (menstrual irregularities) due to hormonal disruption.
- Enamel erosion as a result of acid reflux during vomiting leading to tooth decay and gum disease.
- Dehydration as a result of regular vomiting leading to gastro-intestinal and bowel problems.
- Electrolyte (i.e. sodium and potassium) imbalance which can lead to such as cardiac problems and hypotension (low blood pressure).
- Fainting due to lack of energy.
- Visual indications include swollen glands and bags under the eyes.
- Inflammation of the esophagus.

is a problem they should encourage the client to visit their GP so that either an appropriate counsellor can be found to work with the client in order to advise any treatment or intervention or to seek the GP's consent (for an example GP consent form please visist: www.bloomsbury.com/9781408187234) prior to continuation. For those instructors working within a facility they should identify and make themselves familiar with the policy for managing users with suspected eating disorders.

ENERGY BALANCE

Every individual at some time will experience either weight gain or weight loss. Although a complex topic with many factors that can affect the outcome, it can be explained simply by using something known as the 'energy balance equation' which describes the balance between energy intake (in the form of food) and energy expenditure (in terms of energy stores used for normal function and activity) on a daily basis. Figure 12.2 shows how energy in and energy out can balance or outweigh one another. For example, over the period of a day if the amount of energy taken in is greater than the amount of energy expended then it is likely that the excess energy will result in weight gain.

If weight gain is as a result of a lack of activity or an excess of calories, then there are many adverse health effects associated with this. Conversely if the amount of energy taken in is less than the amount of energy expended, then this could result in weight loss. Too much weight loss can also result in adverse health effects.

Energy in and energy out can be estimated in units of calories. If a client's energy in and out has been estimated and has been found to be too low, appropriate goals could be set to rectify this situation.

ESTIMATING ENERGY OUTPUT

The more appropriate term 'energy expenditure' refers to the amount of energy (calories) we use and is calculated on a daily basis. In very simplistic terms, the more we keep sedentary activities to a minimum the more the energy expenditure will be. There are many methods used to calculate this, but some are not easily accessible such as calorimetry which involves the individual being inside an insulated chamber which measures the amount of heat given off (which is then calculated as calories). One of the most practical methods available to the instructor is the 'ABC method', where estimating total energy expenditure (TEE) can be done by following steps A to C of the example

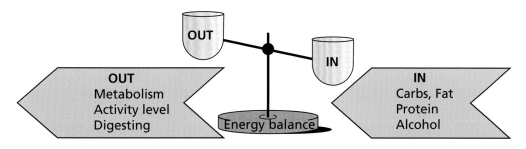

Figure 12.2 The energy balance equation

ESTIMATED TEE RECORD SHEET

STEP A

A – Active Metabolic Rate
Select one of the options depending on whether the level of daily exercise for the client is classed as Inactive, Moderately Active or Very Active:

Inactive		Moderately Active		Very Active	
Male	Female	Male	Female	Male	Female
1.4	1.4	1.7	1.6	1.9	1.8

STEP B

B – Basal Metabolic Rate (measured in Kilocalories-Kcals).
Multiply the figure in step A by the BMR found in the table below recommended by the DoH:

Age range	Males	Females
10 – 17 yr	$(17.7 \times W) + 657$	$(13.4 \times W) + 692$
18 – 29 yr	$(15.1 \times W) + 692$	$(14.8 \times W) + 487$
30 – 59 yr	$(11.5 \times W) + 873$	$(8.3 \times W) + 846$
60 – 74 yr	$(11.9 \times W) + 700$	$(9.2 \times W) + 687$
75+ yr	$(8.4 \times W) + 821$	$(9.8 \times W) + 624$

W = weight in kg.

STEP C

C – Consumption of food – the digestion of food requires a certain amount of energy to do so, therefore, add an extra 10% of the total from steps A and B. Therefore:
Total energy expenditure = Step A x Step B + 10%

Client name   Date

Step A =   Step B =   A X B =   + 10% =

TEE = ...Kcals

Figure 12.3 Estimated TEE record sheet (for a blank template visit: www.bloomsbury.com/9781408187234).

recording sheet in figure 12.3, which breaks down TEE into three main areas:

A = Active metabolic rate (AMR) – which is the amount of energy needed over and above a sedentary level.

B = Basal metabolic rate (BMR) – which is the rate at which the body uses energy at rest and is measured in Kilocalories.

C = Consumption of food – which is the calories needed to digest food.

ESTIMATING ENERGY INPUT

Energy input refers to how much we eat (measured in calories) and involves the complicated process of collecting nutritional information from the client. As with all methods of collecting client data it is essential that confidentiality is addressed in both collecting and storing the information.

The purpose of this information is to estimate the energy intake for comparison against the energy expenditure in order to advise the client in relation to Plate Model advice. Any further analysis of the diet is beyond the scope of the personal trainer and as such the Code of Ethics states that the client be referred to a more qualified person: a Registered Dietician for those who are wanting a general healthy eating diet or an accredited Sports Dietician for those who have specific performance goals. Information is normally gathered by the use of diaries but be aware that individuals often do not keep accurate records and tend to underestimate what they have actually consumed, therefore, work closely with clients when first using this method. The minimum time recommended for keeping a food diary is at least 3–7 days to allow enough information to be assessed, and especially over the weekend as

dietary habits are often different in this period. Figure 12.4 lays out all the information necessary to keep a successful food diary, although there are others available too.

When interpreting a food diary it is crucial to have as much detailed information as possible. Make sure that the client notes down the following:

- Remember to include snacks
- How was the food cooked i.e. fried, boiled, grilled
- Don't forget sauces and spreads such as cream, tomato based and butter
- Include alcohol as this has calories
- Detail i.e. what exactly was in a salad and what type of milk was used on cereal

In order to estimate the average daily calorie intake, the calorie content of the foods eaten must be recorded in the food diary for each twenty-four-hour period. For this reason it is important to get the client to keep all the labels from food wrappers and containers – or perhaps to record this information using the camera on their smartphone – as this often contains nutritional information such as energy in Kilocalories. This is not always possible especially when using fresh produce, therefore, use one of the many websites that offer information on the energy content of specific food items. There will always be errors in this type of estimation as not all software is developed using evidence based knowledge (and could be biased by suppliers who sponsor the software). However, the main point of doing this exercise with the client is to generally assess the quality of the diet in terms of appropriate amounts of energy (the majority in the form of carbohydrate) and a balance across the food groups in the plate model.

DAILY FOOD DIARY

Time of Day	Food or Fluid Consumed	Food group	Amount (g) or Portion Size	Kilocals
Morning				
Midday				
Evening				
			Total Kcals =	

Client name   Date

Activity level

Figure 12.4 Typical daily food diary (for a blank template please visit: www.bloomsbury.com/9781408187234).

ANALYSING NUTRITIONAL INFORMATION

13

THE NOS LEVEL 3 PERSONAL TRAINER CRITERIA COVERED IN THIS CHAPTER ARE:

- The legal and ethical implications of collecting nutritional information
- An understanding of basic dietary assessment methods
- How to apply the principles of goal setting when offering nutritional advice
- Barriers which may prevent clients achieving their nutritional goals
- When to involve people other than the client in nutritional goal setting
- Formats for recording information in a way that will help you to interpret and analyse
- The importance of safeguarding the collected nutritional information and how to do so
- How to obtain clients' informed consent before you begin collecting nutritional information
- How to identify and agree nutritional goals and translate them into basic healthy eating advice that reflects current national guidelines
- How to analyse and interpret collected information to identify clients' needs and nutritional goals in comparison to national guidelines/the national food model
- An understanding of the information that needs to be collected to be able to safely and effectively offer nutritional advice to clients
- How to apply basic motivational strategies to encourage healthy eating and prevent noncompliance or relapse
- The range of professionals and professional bodies involved in the area of nutrition
- Different methods that can be used to measure body composition and health risk in relation to weight:
  - Body Mass Index (BMI)
  - Waist circumference (WC)
  - Waist-to-hip ratio
  - Skin folds and skin fold indices
  - Bioelectrical impedance

- How to interpret information gained from methods used to assess body composition and health risk in relation to weight (use of 'norms')
- How to sensitively divulge collected information and 'results' to clients
- The needs for reappraisal of client's body composition and other relevant health parameters at agreed stages of the programme

INFORMATION GATHERING AND GOAL SETTING

Regardless of the method used to collect nutritional information, nutritional goals should be set based upon the information given by the client and after the trainer has discussed their goals with them. Because of the nature of the information to be collected it is advisable to gain written consent from the client that they understand the sensitive nature of the information they might divulge and that the information will be used to set individual nutritional goals. The 'informed consent' as it is better known should also state that information will be dealt with in a confidential manner but certain information might be better dealt with by more qualified persons, therefore, discussions regarding referral might take place (for an example informed consent form please visit: www.bloomsbury.com/9781408187234).

As with exercise goals the SMART principle can be applied to nutritional goals in order to give a greater chance of success. Also, goals should be identified that are short, medium and long term in order to identify if the programme is successful or needs to modified in the future. Goals should always be discussed with the client, however, it may also be important to involve those close to the client in this process as they often have a direct influence on eating behaviour (though be aware that others may not wish to

become involved). The nutritional goals record sheet in figure 13.1 is a useful tool to help instructors analyse nutritional information and set goals. The template includes an option to record the energy in and out. Energy in should be based on calculating the average energy over the period of one week of food diaries collected from the client (i.e. total energy from 7 days ÷ 7). Energy out should be in relation to that particular week. From the information in the collected food diaries the trainer should also be able to estimate (in approximate percentage terms) the amount of food from each plate model group and record this in the nutritional goals template. Trainers could set the food group goals based on the plate model guidance but taking into account any further requirements of exercise.

The template allows for goals to be set so that the client has a clear understanding of what the nutritional goals are and also provides an accu-

Tip

As with all confidential information that trainers gather it is subject to the Data Protection Act 1998 (www.legislation.gov.uk) and as such trainers should make themselves aware of the regulations relating to the storage and usage of such information.

NUTRITIONAL GOALS RECORD SHEET

Client name   Date

Body fat %

Energy in (weekly average) in Kcals   Energy out (TEE) in Kcals

Energy balance (Kcals in − Kcals out)

Targets	Actual	Goal

Estimate the weekly contribution of the following food groups:
• Bread, cereals, potatoes
• Fruit and veg
• Milk and dairy
• Meat and fish
• Fat and sugar

Number of days five small meals/snacks consumed

Number of days alcohol was consumed

Number of days 5 glasses of water consumed

Other specific goals:

Goals NOT achieved this week:

Reason why goal(s) not achieved:

Agreed strategy:

Figure 13.1 Nutritional goals record sheet (for a blank template visit: www.bloomsbury.com/9781408187234).

rate record for instructors to identify the success of the programme in relation to the goals. It is important that the client be encouraged to reflect each week (or whatever short-term period is agreed) as to the success in relation to agreed goals. Those goals that were not achieved (due to perceived barriers), could be recorded on the example record sheet in figure 13.1 and strategies put in place for the forthcoming period in order to overcome the perceived barriers.

Table 13.1 Common strategies for nutritional goals

Nutritional goals	Common strategies
• Fat content – less than 30% of total intake. • Saturated fat – less than 10% of total.	• Choose skimmed milk over full-fat. • Try to grill rather than fry and trim the meat. • Chose low fat options and spread thinly on bread. • Avoid snacks such as biscuits, cakes and pastries which are high in fat. • Vegetable oil rather than solid fat (lard).
• Carbs – 55–60% of total intake. • Simple carbs – less than 10%.	• Try to include veg in every meal. • Snack on a variety of fruits. • Make the largest proportion of a meal the veg and not the protein. • Chose multi-grain type breads and cereals. • Avoid sugary drinks. Choose water.
• Protein – 10–15%.	• Eat a variety of sources and try to include non animal sources. • Trim the fat of any meat. • Reduce the amount of red meat. • Include oily fish.
• Salt – no more than 3–6g per day.	• Do not add table salt to any food. • Try to avoid processed foods. • Avoid salted snacks. • Read the labels!
• Fibre – 30g per day.	• Eat fruit and veg every day. • Dried fruits can be used as snacks. • Choose whole wheat or wholegrain options (bread, pasta, cereal). • Include beans and pulses in your diet.
• Dietary cholesterol – less than 300mg per day.	• Limit intake of eggs. • Only eat liver, heart, kidney, etc., occasionally.
• Alcohol – limit to 1 or 2 drinks per day	• Stick to guideline levels or less. • Choose low or non-alcoholic substitutes. • Drink water before alcohol to give the feeling of being full.

NUTRITIONAL BARRIERS

Nutritional goals are similar to exercise goals in that they both require the client to undergo a process of change (see behavioural change, chapter 3). Identifying which stage the client may be at, however, is complex so it is advised that trainers simply discuss the readiness to change with their clients in relation to any nutritional goals that may have been agreed.

As changing people's behaviours in regard to nutrition is difficult, and often requires a degree of training, trainers are advised to follow general guidelines when recommending a nutrition plan based on the nutritional goals record sheet. Table 13.1 gives a list of common nutritional goals that are in line with government guidelines and a selection of typical nutritional strategies that will help to achieve the goals.

It is important to set small goals and progress when they are achieved rather than try to initiate a complete lifestyle change from the start. As larger changes are more likely to fail it is better to set goals that can be achieved in order to give the client a feeling of success which should have a positive effect on adherence to any programme. Reminding the client on a regular basis about the reasons they want to achieve their goals should help to motivate them and also adapt them if necessary.

BODY COMPOSITION

On the nutritional goals record sheet, there is an option to record the body fat percentage of the client. This is useful as it can help the trainer gauge the success of the programme (both exercise and nutritional) in relation to the agreed goals of the client. In simple terms, body composition can be thought of as the amount of fat and lean tissue within the body. It is generally accepted that body fat percentage can influence both athletic performance and increase an individual's risk of disease. The term obesity is used to describe an individual who is carrying excess bodyweight in relation to their height or an individual who has excessive amounts of body fat, which has been shown to increase the risk of disease such as hypertension, type 2 diabetes and coronary heart disease and reduce life expectancy.

METHODS OF TESTING BODY COMPOSITION

Measuring body composition is a complicated issue as the only 'direct' way to measure true body composition is by dissection of cadavers to see how much fat tissue there is. All other methods (see table 13.2 for a selection of the most common methods) of testing for body composition are based on estimates made from the few cadaver studies that have been carried out over the years and are known as 'indirect' methods. Many of these methods are unavailable to the trainer (densitometry, plethysmography and body imaging) as the equipment is prohibitively expensive and also is required to be carried out in a clinical environment. Several universities, however, have such specialist equipment and instructors who have a relationship with the university might be allowed access for testing purposes. Most trainers, however, use methods such as bio-electrical impedance and anthropometry.

Whatever the method used, having tested for body composition it is useful to have data against which to make comparison. Data such as this is known as 'normative data' and is usually available in table format. Essentially, this is information relating to specific tests (in this case

Table 13.2 Indirect methods of measuring body composition

Method	Description
Densitometry	For example, underwater weighing. The measurement of density is based on the Archimedes' principle that 'a body immersed in a fluid is balanced by a buoyancy force equivalent to the weight of fluid displaced'. By measuring weight when submerged, a measure of an individual's body density can be found and converted to body fat percentage.
Plethysmography)	This is measured by the amount of air displaced by the body, which is a similar principle to that of Archimedes. A person sits in a small chamber and the volume of air displaced is used to calculate body fat percentage.
Body-imaging techniques	Dual-energy X-ray absorptiometry (DXA) and Nuclear Magnetic Resonance imaging (NMR) are known as body imaging techniques. DXA works through analysing the passing of X-rays with low energy and high energy through the body. The passing of these X-rays depends on the composition of the tissues it passes through. NMR uses powerful magnetic fields, which provide a clearer picture of soft tissues than X-rays do.
Bio-electrical impedance	Body Stat and other similar electrical devices are in this category. It is based on the principle that an electric current flows easier through water than fat so depending on the current flow body fat percentage can be calculated.
Anthropometry	Skin-fold, height, body weight, girths (such as waist circumference and waist-to-hip ratio), bone widths, and BMI. For skin-fold measurements, callipers are used to measure the amount of fat at various sites on the body.

body composition) which has been collected from thousands of subjects in order to produce common population guidelines such as those published by the World Health Organisation as can be seen in table 13.3.

Methods such as electrical impedance and skinfolds that give results in body fat percentage can be compared directly to such norm tables but it should be noted that these are very general guidelines and should be treated as such.

There are, however, methods of testing body composition other than measuring body fat percentage. For example, the Body Mass Index (BMI), which is an index of risk of developing associated disease (as mentioned previously). Body Mass Index is a very common method that simply divides a person's weight by their height squared (height multiplied by height) to give a score in units of kg/m^2.

Body Mass Index formula:

BMI = Weight (kg) ÷ Height (m) squared

Table 13.3 Age-adjusted body fat percentage recommendations

WOMEN

Age	Underfat	Healthy Range	Overweight	Obese
20–40 yrs	Under 21%	21–33%	33–39%	Over 39%
41–60 yrs	Under 23%	23–35%	35–40%	Over 40%
61–79 yrs	Under 24%	24–36%	36–42%	Over 42%

MEN

Age	Underfat	Healthy Range	Overweight	Obese
20–40 yrs	Under 8%	8–19%	19–25%	Over 25%
41–60 yrs	Under 11%	11–2 2%	22–27%	Over 27%
61–79 yrs	Under 13%	13–25%	25–30%	Over 30%

If the trainer chooses to use this method, then they should compare the results against published 'norms'; for instance, the National Institute for Health and Clinical Excellence (NICE) guidelines of 200. As can be seen in table 13.4. A BMI of less than 18.5 is considered to be underweight which, like being overweight, can have adverse health consequences. A BMI of 18.5 up to 24.9 is considered to be low risk (healthy weight) whereas a BMI of 25 to 29.9 is classed as overweight, and 30 or above is classed as obese (sub-divided into three classes). It should be noted that this method has been shown to be inaccurate for those individuals who are considered to be muscular or athletic, women who are pregnant or breast-feeding or individuals who are classed as being frail.

There are also other methods of assessing risk such as waist circumference measurements and waist-to-hip ratio. By simply dividing the waist measurement by the hip measurement a ratio can be found which can be compared to norms (such as those published by the World Health

Table 13.4 BMI classifications according to NICE guidelines

Classification	BMI (kg/m^2)
Underweight	Less than 18.5
Healthy weight	18.5–24.9
Overweight	25–29.9
Obesity class I	30–34.9
Obesity class II	35–39.9
Obesity class III	40 or more

Table 13.5	Risk categories for waist-to-hip ratio scores				
Gender	**Age**	**Low Risk**	**Moderate Risk**	**High Risk**	**Very High Risk**
Men	20–29	<0.83	0.83–0.88	0.89–0.94	>0.94
	30–39	<0.84	0.84–0.91	0.92–0.96	>0.96
	40–49	<0.88	0.88–0.95	0.96–1.00	>1.00
	50–59	<0.90	0.90–0.96	0.97–1.02	>1.02
	60–69	<0.91	0.91–0.98	0.99–1.03	>1.03
Women	20–29	<0.71	0.71–0.77	0.78–0.82	>0.82
	30–39	<0.72	0.72–0.78	0.79–0.84	>0.84
	40–49	<0.73	0.73–0.79	0.80–0.87	>0.87
	50–59	<0.74	0.74–0.81	0.82–0.88	>0.88
	60–69	<0.76	0.76–0.83	0.84–0.90	>0.90

Organization in table 13.5) in order to identify a risk classification. This is quite a common method, even though it has been criticised due to being dependent on the structure of the pelvis and muscle distribution as well as needing two measurements which can increase the risk of error.

Another method that is generally considered to be more accurate is by measuring waist circumference, which is also thought to be a reasonable indication of the risk of certain diseases such as Type 2 diabetes and coronary heart disease. Taking only one measurement can also be easier for the subject to remember and focus on as opposed to having to remember two different measurements. Table 13.6 shows the waist circumference risk table adapted from the ACSM.

Some other guidelines go even further than using just one method to assess the risk of health problems associated with obesity. For example, the NICE guidelines on prevention, identification, assessment and management of overweight and obese in adults and children (see http://www.nice.org.uk/cg43) suggest that the risk of the associated health problems should be identified using a combination of BMI and waist circumference for those people with a BMI of less than 35 kg/m². This is because for adults with a BMI of 35kg/m² or more, it is assumed that the risks are very high regardless of the waist circumference measurement. Table 13.7 shows the category of risk calculated from the combination of BMI and waist circumference measurements.

Table 13.6 Risk categories for waist circumference scores

Risk	Men cm	Men inches	Women cm	Women inches
Very High	>120	>47	>110	>43.5
High	100–120	39.5–47	90–109	35.5–43
Low	80–99	31.5–39	70–89	28.5–35
Very Low	<80	<31.5	<70	< 28.5

Table 13.7 NICE risk categories for BMI and waist circumference

	Waist circumference Low	Waist circumference High	Waist circumference Very high
Male	< 94cm	94cm–102cm	> 102cm
Female	< 80cm	80cm–88cm	> 88cm
Normal weight	No increased risk	No increased risk	Increased risk
Overweight (BMI 25 to 29.9)	No increased risk	Increased risk	High risk
Obesity 1 (BMI 30 to 34.9)	Increased risk	High risk	Very high risk

PART SEVEN
HEALTH AND SAFETY IN PRACTICE

HEALTH, SAFETY AND WELFARE

THE NOS LEVEL 3 PERSONAL TRAINER CRITERIA COVERED IN THIS CHAPTER ARE:

- The values or codes of practice relevant to the work you are carrying out
- The requirements for health, safety and welfare that are relevant to your work
- Manufacturers' guidelines and instructions for the use of facilities and equipment
- Why health, safety and welfare are important in a sport and activity environment
- The persons responsible for health and safety in your workplace
- Your organisation's security procedures

Due to the very nature of physical activity and exercise it is important for trainers to understand that they will encounter many health and safety issues on an almost daily basis, and so it is important to be aware of the issues surrounding them. This is not just because of the emerging litigational environment that they work in, but, more importantly, for the safety of themselves and their clients. As with all recommended guidelines in relation to health and safety, they are based on certain laws, of which the trainer should be aware.

SOURCES OF ENGLISH LAW

There are three main sources of law in the English legal system:

- Statute law and delegated legislation
- Common law and precedent
- European Community law (EC law)

Statute law and delegated legislation

Also commonly referred to as 'Acts of Parliament' or 'legislation', statute law is simply law that is passed by parliament. An example of this would be the Health and Safety at Work Act 1974 (www.hse.gov. uk). The term 'delegated legislation' is law made by bodies to which parliament has delegated its law-making power. An example of this would be the Management of Health and Safety at Work Regulations 1999 (www.hse.gov.uk), which is essentially a more detailed set of regulations relating to specific sections of the Health and Safety at Work Act 1974.

Common law and precedent

The term common law, or 'case law' as it is otherwise known, refers to law passed by court judges that is based on other previous similar cases. With regards to common law, trainers should make themselves aware of something known as 'tort law'. The word 'tort' (in Scotland known as 'delict') is derived from an old French word for a wrong doing. Tort law deals with situations where a person's behaviours or actions (not necessarily illegal) have unfairly caused someone to suffer loss or harm. In other words, trainers have a duty of care when working with clients to keep them safe. This is clearly important within the sport and fitness environments.

European Community law (EC law)

The third source known as European Community law was first established in the UK following the birth of the European Economic Community (EEC) in 1973. Many laws now include provision to take account of European law.

HEALTH AND SAFETY AT WORK

As in any work environment, the area of health and safety is an important issue for trainers, especially when putting together clients' exercise programmes. The statutory framework relating to health and safety (and to risk management) is, in the main part, covered by the Management of Health and Safety at Work Regulations (MHSW) 1999 and the Health and Safety at Work Act (HSWA) 1974.

THE MANAGEMENT OF HEALTH AND SAFETY AT WORK REGULATIONS 1999

The MHSW essentially outlines the role of the employer (trainers whose business employs one or more PTs) and the self-employed (self-employed PTs).

Employers

All employers shall make suitable and sufficient assessment of:

a – risks to the health and safety of employees to which they are exposed at work; and

b – the risks to the health and safety of persons (not employees) in connection with the conduct of employees.

Self-employed

All self-employed persons shall make suitable and sufficient assessment of:

a – the risks to their own health and safety to which they are exposed at work; and

b – the risks to the health and safety of persons in connection with their conduct.

In other words, the act is suggesting that it is necessary for trainers to regularly carry out a formal risk assessment in relation to employees and clients (see page 213).

THE HEALTH AND SAFETY AT WORK ACT 1974

The HSWA covers broad principles such as the role of employers and self-employed people, as well as those appointed persons for all areas of health and safety, in relation to prevention of accidents. Although the HSWA is an extensive document, the most relevant sections for the trainer include those in table 14.1.

In other words the trainer has a duty of care during their work with regards to their own

Table 14.1	**Relevant section synopses from the HSWA 1974**
Section	**Overview**
1	This section outlines the duty of employers to ensure the broad provisions that the health and safety of all people are protected from risks including the control of hazardous substances.
2	This section deals with the general duties of employers related to the health, safety and welfare of all employees. This includes system maintenance, training, supervision and the provision of relevant procedures.
3	This section relates to the general duties of employers and self-employed to clients in terms of risks to health and safety and information to make clients aware of this.
4	This section mainly deals with the safety of equipment used within certain premises.
7	This section relates to the general duties of employees taking care of the health and safety of themselves and others.

health and safety as well as that of their clients. Larger health and fitness organisations should, by law, make a health and safety policy statement available to all staff and provide employees with relevant training. However, prior to working in any health and fitness environment, the trainer must make themselves familiar with several fundamental safety issues in the workplace and be aware of procedures that could help to minimise the occurrence of accident or injury as inevitably this will occur. If trainers do not make appropriate efforts to minimise the risk and injury does occur, then it could be classed as 'negligence'. The very nature of physical activity means that it can never be 100% risk free, therefore, as long as trainers do what is reasonable to make people safe then there will be little chance of successful negligence claims (the Compensation Act, 2006 gives a full explanation relating to negligence legislation).

If the trainer is self-employed, then they are directly responsible for any negligent act, however, if the trainer is employed while a negligent act is committed then the employer is said to be 'vicariously liable' and as such responsible for the act. Problems do occur, however, in establishing whether trainers are employees or contractors, therefore, it is in the interest of the trainer to identify and familiarise themselves with a variety of policies and procedures that facilities should have if they intend to use a particular facility for instruction purposes. These would include:

- **Normal Operating Procedures (NOPs):** this often includes such things as security procedures and day-to-day operations.
- **Emergency Operating Procedures (EOPs):** such as fire and medical emergency.
- **Security procedures:** all facilities should have

procedures relating to the 24-hour security of the facility itself.

- **Young Persons Safety Act 1995 (www.legislation.gov.uk):** to make provision for the regulation of centres and providers of facilities where children and young persons under the age of 18 engage in adventure activities, including provision for the imposition of requirements relating to safety.
- **Manual Handling Operations Regulations 2004 (www.hse.gov.uk):** this outlines risk assessment procedures for manual handling.
- **Control of Substances Hazardous to Health Regulations 2002 (www.hse.gov.uk):** this is the law that requires employers to control substances that are hazardous to health and gives advice on how to prevent or reduce workers' exposure to hazardous substances.
- **Manufacturers' guidelines and instructions:** most facilities employ the use of equipment that will outline usage guidelines. Even though it is the responsibility of the facility to adhere to these guidelines it is always advisable that trainers be aware of the guidelines relating to the equipment or space within the facility that they use.

If a trainer is unsure in any way, they should consult the relevant person in order to clarify the issue. This is also the case should a trainer feel that procedures do not reflect health and safety regulations in any way. The environment, be it a National Governing Body or public/private fitness centre, should provide all employees with the relevant procedures relating to the policies mentioned.

Tip

Trainers should make sure that they have made all policies and procedures accessible to clients. A website is often the most useful place for doing this so that clients can be directed to the site to view any policies or procedures that they are interested in. If the trainer is working on behalf of an employer, the client should be directed to the employer's source of policies and procedures.

PROTECTION OF CHILDREN AND THE VULNERABLE

15

THE NOS LEVEL 3 PERSONAL TRAINER CRITERIA COVERED IN THIS CHAPTER ARE:

- What is safeguarding and protecting the welfare of children and vulnerable adults?
- Your own role and responsibilities for safeguarding and protecting children and vulnerable adults
- The range of types of abuse: physical, emotional, neglect and sexual
- The basic indicators and impact of abuse: physical, emotional, neglect and sexual
- The risks that individual or potential abusers pose to children and vulnerable adults
- Your organisation's policies and procedures in relation to safeguarding and protecting, including the reporting procedures
- What to do if you have concerns about possible abuse
- How to respond to a child or someone else disclosing abuse or concerns about abuse
- What you should do if there are barriers to reporting your concerns
- Statutory agencies with responsibilities for safeguarding and protecting, and when and how you should contact them
- Why it is important to share concerns about possible abuse with others
- The limits of your own competence in regard to safeguarding and protecting and why it is important to involve others
- Why it is important to treat information about possible abuse confidentially
- The importance of client care both to the client and the organisation
- Why it is important to deal effectively with client/individual needs
- The types of information which clients usually need
- How to respond to requests according to the organisations procedures
- Where to source relevant information to meet client needs

CHILD AND VULNERABLE ADULT PROTECTION

According to Her Majesty's Government, any adult who works with children has a responsibility (known as duty of care) to keep children safe and protect them from sexual, physical and emotional harm. Failure to do this could be regarded as neglect and could lead to prosecution.

Key aspects of legislation have recently been extended to include similar standards of protection to 'vulnerable adults'. A vulnerable adult is defined by the UK government as 'a person aged 18 years or over who is in receipt or need of community care services by reason of mental or other disability, age or illness and who is unable to take care of themselves or protect themselves against significant harm or exploitation'. A vulnerable client on the other hand can be described as someone undergoing a 'special' physiological process that puts them at a greater risk of an exercise-related event (e.g. childhood, ageing and pregnancy). In the health and fitness industry, the term 'special population' is often used to describe a vulnerable client.

'Duty of care' (which falls under the 'law of tort' in England or 'delict' in Scotland) essentially means that any trainer working in the industry must be aware that they must exercise a reasonable level of care in order to avoid injury to individuals and their property.

In 1999 the Protection of Children Act was implemented with a view to increase the level of protection for children by screening those wishing to supervise children. People deemed unsuitable would be those whose names appeared on the following lists:

- List 99 from The Department of Education And Skills (DfES).
- Protection of Children Act list.
- Protection of Vulnerable Adult list.
- Department of Health list.

Anyone wishing to work with children is required have their name cross-referenced with lists such as those above. Since November 2012, an organisation within the Home Office called the Disclosures and Barring services deals with the checks (See http://www.homeoffice.gov.uk/agencies-public-bodies/dbs/about-us1/what-we-do/before-the-dbs/).

Most businesses that employ trainers will have in place procedures to ensure that unsuitable people are prevented from working with children and vulnerable adults. Facilities should make their policies on safeguarding children and vulnerable adults available to all employees so it is in the interest of the trainer to identify these policies as they can also give guidance on how to protect the trainer from potential accusation. Self-employed trainers, however, have a responsibility to make sure this is done (for more information on this process please visit the following websites: www.disclosure.gov.uk or www.crb.gov.uk). The Joint Chief Inspectors' Report on Arrangements to Safeguard Children (2002) is also a useful text for trainers. Safeguarding and protection of children and vulnerable adults covers many areas that the trainer should be aware of such as physical contact, confidentiality, sexual conduct, social contact, communication and comforting as outlined in table 15.1

PHYSICAL CONTACT

There are situations in which physical contact may be necessary from a teaching perspective. Those clients who are vulnerable can sometimes

Table 15.1 Summary of areas of duty of care

Area	Main points	Advice	Information
Confidentiality	• Treat all information as confidential. • Do not allow others access to this information.	• Keep confidential information in a lockable place.	Data Protection Act 1998
Sexual conduct	• ALL sexual activity is a criminal offence. • Special attention can be construed as grooming. • Report any concerns about infatuation.	• Never make sexual remarks or jokes. • Never discuss your own relationship. • Always make contact by email or phone through the parent or guardian. • Avoid having favourites and giving special attention.	Sexual Offences Act 2003 Working Together to Safeguard Children: 2006 HM Government
Social contact	• Social contact between trainers and vulnerable clients is not encouraged. • Trainers should never invite vulnerable clients to their homes.	• Make supervisors aware of any social contact with vulnerable clients and their families. • Never allow vulnerable clients into your home without their parents.	
Communication	• This includes phones, emails, websites and cameras. • Contact only in professional instances such as informing that sessions are cancelled.	• Always communicate through the parent or guardian. • Always get written permission for photos or videos.	Code of Conduct.
Physical contact	• Physical contact is often required in instructing as long as it is appropriate. • Some vulnerable clients may feel uncomfortable by this whereas others may initiate inappropriate contact. • There may be cultural or religious issues.	• Get permission from vulnerable clients before any contact. • Try to keep parents informed of the need for this contact in instructing. • Make sure vulnerable clients know of the boundaries. • Report any issues immediately.	Code of Conduct.

Table 15.1	Summary of areas of duty of care (*cont.*)		
Area	**Main points**	**Advice**	**Information**
Comforting	• Vulnerable clients often become distressed for many reasons especially younger children. • Some vulnerable clients may use this to seek comfort. • Professional judgement is key.	• Often a hand on the shoulder is enough to comfort. • Never comfort on a one-to-one situation unless another trainer or parent is present. • Record any issues you may be unsure about.	

feel uncomfortable with physical contact. It's good practice for the trainer to always ask first if it is all right to do so and explain to the client the purpose and what they are going to do. For instance, the grip of a barbell might need to be adjusted so the trainer will need to make contact with the hand and wrist of the client in order to make the adjustment. Trainers should be professional in the way they do this and never appear to be secretive or dwell in any way. It is often good practice to inform parents in advance of what the intention is in terms of instruction (especially for very young children) so they understand the potential need for the contact.

Unfortunately, it is sometimes the case (especially with those who have suffered abuse themselves) that individuals may seek inappropriate contact with the trainer. Regardless of the circumstances, any situation where a vulnerable person initiates inappropriate contact should be dealt with. The trainer needs to make the boundaries clear (in a sensitive way) but then report this to a senior person as soon as possible. In order to minimise the risk of any inappropriate situation developing (or being misconstrued by others as developing), trainers should try to minimise phys-ical contact as best as possible. However, there are situations where contact cannot be avoided. For example:

- Demonstrating the use of certain equipment
- Helping to tie shoelaces
- Providing a steadying hand on performance of an exercise technique

In these situations it is important that the trainer always maintains a professional approach. The golden rule for trainers is to *never* be left in a one-to-one situation with any vulnerable person. If a situation arises where a vulnerable person is waiting for parents and only the trainer is present, they should wait in an area where other people are around (for example, in the reception area of the club in which they are instructing).

CONFIDENTIALITY

Trainers often need to gather information about vulnerable clients that is confidential (address, contact details, etc.) and that information must be treated as such at all times. If a trainer is not sure about what information is confidential or how to treat it, they should access a copy of the

Data Protection Act 1998 (www.legislation.gov.uk) which provides all the information relevant to this area.

SEXUAL CONDUCT

The Sexual Offences Act 2003 (www.legislation.gov.uk) in relation to abuse of positions of trust states that where a person aged 18 years of age or over is in a specified position of trust with a child under 18 years of age, it is an offence for that person to engage in any sexual activity with or in the presence of that child, or to cause or incite that child to engage in or watch any sexual activity. There is absolutely no ambiguity about this statement as it means that any sexual activity is a criminal offence! Unfortunately though, it is quite a common occurrence where children become infatuated with their trainers. This is an extremely sensitive situation in which trainers must be highly professional at all times and if a trainer does suspect some kind of infatuation on the part of the client, they must speak with a professional person immediately. Trainers should be especially aware that showing special attention to certain children, regardless of their gender, can sometimes be seen by others as 'grooming'.

SOCIAL CONTACT

In simple terms, trainers should not seek to have any social contact with vulnerable clients or their families. In practice, however, this is not always easy to do as many trainers already have social contact with families before undertaking an instructing role. Even if this is the case, trainers should never allow vulnerable clients in their own home without the presence of their parents or carers.

COMMUNICATION

This area relates to the use of any communication or recording tools such as mobile phones, emails, websites, cameras and videos, etc. Trainers should always be mindful of anything that could be construed as grooming. For instance, personal mobile or home numbers should never be given out and trainers should also be wary of any social networking communication using mediums such as Facebook. Regardless of the medium used, any communication either to or from the trainer should always be done through the parents, carers or guardians.

COMFORTING

It is not uncommon for vulnerable people to become upset for some reason or another. Human instinct to put an arm around the shoulder for the purpose of comfort can be very strong, however, this is not recommended in most cases, especially when working on a one-to-one basis. The trainer should use their professional judgement in each case as the circumstances could be very different. For instance, the person might become upset because they didn't perform well, so a reassuring hand on the shoulder or pat on the back would be enough in this case. In the case of the person falling and hurting themselves, an arm around the shoulder might be needed to console them if they are in a state of distress. The trainer should be aware of any vulnerable person trying to feign distress in order to gain sympathy. If there is a situation that the trainer feels unsure about, they should record the incident and the nature of what happened.

DEALING WITH ABUSE

It is not uncommon for trainers to be approached by a vulnerable client who tells them about an abusive situation involving another trainer or adult. Abuse can take many forms – physical, emotional, neglect, bullying and sexual – and is often difficult to identify especially if the trainer has no previous experience of this type of situation, therefore, trainers should make sure that they understand the nature of each form of abuse.

PHYSICAL ABUSE

This type of abuse is when physical harm is deliberately caused by hitting, burning, biting and shaking, etc., and is characterised by physical injuries that are not explained satisfactorily.

EMOTIONAL ABUSE

This type of abuse relates to persistent situations that have adverse effects on vulnerable peoples' emotional well-being such as constant criticism, sarcasm, bullying and taunting. It also includes situations where the person is made to feel ashamed of any involuntary behaviour they display.

NEGLECT

This is when adults fail to meet a vulnerable person's basic needs (physical, psychological and/or emotional) such as providing protection, food, shelter and affection to the extent that health and development are impaired.

BULLYING

This type of abuse can be verbal, written or physical and can come via the Internet as well. Victims are often shy or sensitive and are usually picked on for being different in some way.

SEXUAL ABUSE

This is when adults (or even other children) use vulnerable people for their own sexual needs.

Contact does not always need to happen as exposure to pornographic material constitutes sexual abuse.

The effects of any form of abuse can be long lasting both physically and psychologically and, quite commonly, the behaviour displayed by children as a result of abuse can persist into adulthood. It is crucial, therefore, that trainers are aware of any signs of abuse, such as:

- Mild to severe pain (acute and chronic) and in some cases injury and even death
- Behavioural problems such as aggression and tantrums
- Development problems (physical, emotional and psychological)
- Learning problems (cognitive and social)
- Self-esteem and self-worth issues
- Withdrawn and introverted behaviour
- Depressive and self-harming tendencies

Recognising signs of abuse can be extremely difficult, therefore, the trainer should be aware of typical signs related to each sub-classification of abuse. Table 15.2 provides an overview of typical physical and behavioural signs but for more information trainers should visit www.nspcc.org.uk or read NSPCC (2000) Child maltreatment in the UK: a study of the prevalence of child abuse and neglect.

Even though reporting any form of abuse can put the trainer in a very delicate situation, it is not the responsibility of the trainer to decide if abuse or inappropriate behaviour has taken place. Cases of false allegation tend to be rare, therefore, immediate action should always be taken. Facilities should have procedures in place for doing so

Table 15.2 Physical and behavioural signs of abuse

Abuse area	Physical signs	Behavioural signs
Physical	Unexplained bruising/hand marks, burns, breaks, scalds	Flinching, covering up, reluctance to see GP Depressed, withdrawn, aggressive outbursts
Emotional	Speech disorders Lack of progress Sudden weight gain or loss	Self-harm, fear of making mistakes Don't take part, strange behaviour Drop in self-esteem
Neglect	Always hungry, underweight Poorly dressed, unclean	Always tired and late Loner, no chaperone
Bullying	Stomach and headaches Scratching and bruising	Mood swings, can't concentrate Poor performance, won't engage, withdrawn
Sexual	Walking discomfort Genital itching Signs of self-harm	Self-harm, no friends, sexual actions Change in behaviour, fear of people Eating problems, having secrets

and it is the responsibility of the trainer to make sure they understand and follow them. In situations where the trainer is not working in or for a facility it is even more important to make sure that procedures are followed, recorded and dealt with in a confidential manner. If a client tries to disclose any form of abuse, the trainer should follow the basic guideline procedures.

1. Stay calm throughout
2. Reassure the person you will take them seriously
3. Explain that you may have to follow a reporting procedure and do not promise anything
4. Encourage the person to tell the whole story but do not probe or ask closed questions (yes, no, etc.)
5. Listen carefully and do not comment on the allegation
6. As soon as possible, record the event and either speak to a colleague for advice or follow reporting procedures

Although this type of incident requires a degree of confidentiality, it is sometimes useful to speak to a qualified and experienced senior colleague about the incident (while keeping anonymity) if the trainer feels that they need help. It may be that the advice is to talk to parents/carers first in order to clarify any concerns. In some situations this might not be appropriate as this could place the vulnerable person at greater risk, and if the trainer feels the case is severe enough, then they should contact either the social services or the police. If the trainer feels that the incident should be reported but the person is in no immediate danger, they should report the incident as soon as possible. When reporting the incident, an example such as that in figure 15.1 could be used. Self-employed, trainers should send their reports (making sure they have a copy for their own records) to the head office of the company they are working under or if independent they

CHILD PROTECTION - INCIDENT REPORT FORM

Name of Child: xxxxxxxxx

Age: 11 years   Date of Birth: xxxxx

Address: 21 Sunshine Avenue, Wilton on Leigh, North Ridingshire

Postcode: NE1 1NE

What happened (in child's own words if possible):

Over a 3-month period I have noticed bruising to the body of xxx and when queried got the same response of 'I fell over'.

When incident happened:

For 3-months since start of programme

Where incident happened:

Was noticed during gym sessions as wearing a vest and bruising was visible.

When was the incident reported:

Today's date

Trainer's observations (i.e. description of behaviour, or injury):

Bruising has been regular to different areas of the back. Behaviour of the child has become more introvert and there is a reluctance on the part of the child to talk about the bruising.

Signed   Date

Figure 15.1 Example child protection incident report form (For a blank template please visist: www.bloomsbury.com/9781408187234)

should contact either SkillsActive or the Register of Exercise Professionals for guidance. If the trainer requires advice for any reason, then they should contact either:

- NSPCC Child Protection Helpline on 0808 8005000; or
- ChildLine on 0800 1111

RISK ASSESSING, INJURIES, ILLNESS AND EMERGENCIES 16

THE NOS LEVEL 3 PERSONAL TRAINER CRITERIA COVERED IN THIS CHAPTER ARE:

- The types of hazards that are likely to occur in your area of work and the accidents and injuries they could cause
- How to identify hazards
- Health, safety and security checks you should follow
- How to carry out basic risk assessments of the types of hazards that may occur
- Why it is important to get advice from a relevant colleague if you are unsure about hazards and risks in your workplace and who you should ask
- How to deal correctly with the types of hazards that may occur in your workplace, taking account of their risks
- Documents relating to health and safety that you may have to complete and how to complete them correctly
- Why you should encourage your colleagues and customers to behave in a safe manner and how to do so
- The importance of making suggestions about health and safety issues and how to do so
- Why it is important to identify and report any differences between health and safety requirements and your workplace's policies and procedures and how to do so
- The types of accidents, injuries and illnesses that may occur in your area of work
- How to respond correctly to emotional distress
- How to deal with these before qualified assistance arrives
- How to decide whether to contact the on-site first aider or immediately call the emergency services
- Who is the on-site first aider and how to contact them
- The procedures you should follow to contact the emergency services
- Why it is important to protect the casualty and others involved from further harm

- The procedures you should follow to protect the casualty and others
- Why it is important to provide comfort and reassurance and how to do so
- Your responsibilities for reporting accidents and the procedures you should follow
- The emergency procedures in your place of work
- What instructions you must give to the people involved
- Your organisation's reporting procedures for emergencies safety and welfare in
- The types of problems that may occur during emergency procedures, why you should report them and who you should report them to

RISK ASSESSMENT

The statutory framework relating to risk management and health and safety at work in the UK is mainly covered by the Management of Health and Safety at Work Regulations (1999) which states that all self-employed persons should carry out risk assessment to identify health and safety risks to clients. All personal training environments have potential hazards and risks and it is the purpose of risk assessment to identify any that might be present.

HAZARDS

Hazards are essentially to do with the environment such as equipment left lying around, ambient temperature not controlled or water spillages on floor surfaces. These types of hazards tend to result in soft tissue injuries such as sprains and strains (see pages 216–17). Substances that are used for cleaning that are not stored or used correctly can also constitute a hazard in terms of breathing in toxic fumes or being exposed to corrosive materials. In this case there is guidance in the form of Control of Substances Hazardous to Health Regulations which all facilities should have.

RISKS

A risk is usually taken to mean a risk to personnel such as the client or trainer. Certain exercises constitute a risk in terms of injury or disability, and usually the risk is larger or greater depending on the individual. Although risks cannot be eradicated completely, they can be recognised, addressed and minimised. When planning an exercise session, it is advisable to complete and document a risk assessment for all environments even though there is no legal obligation to do so if an organisation has less than five employees. Getting into the habit of doing this acts as a written reminder for the trainer as well as providing evidence that preventative steps were taken, should an accident occur. In practical terms this simply means thinking about any possible risks that there might be and strategies to make them less so. Often a good place to start is by asking questions about the planned activity. Table 16.1 gives a typical scenario response to general risk questions.

Each question would then need a risk rating of low, medium or high. What actually constitutes a low, medium or high risk situation might be slightly different depending on how individual trainers perceive each situation. Whatever the

Table 16.1 Risk assessment questions

	Question	Scenario response
1	Are there any potential hazards which might result in significant harm?	Speed ladders used for sprint drills.
2	Who might be harmed and how?	The trainer or the clients. The use of speed ladders could result in tripping and injury caused by falling.
3	Is the risk of significant harm low/unlikely, medium/possible or high/probable?	Medium.
4	Where the risk is identified as medium or high, has an action been identified?	Only use the ladders on grass to lessen the impact on falling. Only allow one person at a time in the ladder. Do not run backwards through the ladder.

trainer's perception of the rating of a situation, the following guidelines could be adopted:

- LOW RISK – further precautions are optional and the activity can go ahead.
- MEDIUM RISK – further precautions should be taken before the activity proceeds.
- HIGH RISK – the risk should be reduced before running the activity.

If there are medium or high risks associated with the session, then a risk assessment must be carried out. There are many types of risk assessment forms that can be used but figure 16.1 (for a template visit: www.bloomsbury.com/9781408187234) can be used to help formulate and document a basic risk assessment.

HEALTH AND SAFETY CHECKS

As well as carrying out a risk assessment prior to each session it is advisable to get into the habit of performing health and safety checks before each session and also documenting this in case of any potential future problems. There is no definitive checklist for this as all environments differ slightly and each requires a different format. Figure 16.1 gives an example of some of the areas that might be included so that the trainer can check each area prior to the start of the session. For example, checking the environment would require the trainer to make sure that wherever the session takes place it is suitable in terms of flooring, space, temperature, etc. When checking equipment, whatever is being used for the session should be checked that it is working properly. Facilities should have manufacturers' guidelines on how to maintain equipment available to its staff. (Maintenance logs should also be kept accessible.) In terms of screening, it is always advisable to carry out a verbal screening check prior to the start of each session as clients might have been injured or become ill since you last saw them. As part of all pre-session safety briefs, trainers should always reinforce the importance of

EXAMPLE RISK ASSESSMENT FORM

Venue: Gym   Date of check:

Trainer: Session: Circuit and weights

Potential Risk	Lo Med Hi	Method of minimising risk	Action to be taken	✓
Participant recovering from shoulder injury.	Med	Limit range of motion and weight.	Set pec dec range to start at limited range of motion.	✓
Participants could run into walls in indoor venue.	Med	Limit running area.	Use cones to set the limits of the session away from the walls.	✓
Participants might have to wait if machines busy. Could cool down.	Lo	Give alternative exercise in programme.	Have cards with alternatives for this scenario.	✓

                                                                        Yes   No

Environment:

Suitable clothing:

Emergency points:

First Aid kit:

Telephone:

Water:

Equipment:

Screening:

Issues:

Details:

Signed: Date:

First Aider Name: Contact:

Figure 16.1 Example of a typical risk assessment form

acting in a safe manner throughout the duration of any session. The trainer should always lead by example in terms of their behaviour and participation within the session. If any issues relating to health and safety do arise, however, then they could be noted on the risk assessment form as a record and also as an action to be dealt with prior to any further sessions.

HEALTH AND SAFETY POLICIES/ PROCEDURES

Whatever the range of health and safety checks that the trainer decides upon, if working within an organisation, it is useful to identify and familiarise yourself with the organisation's policies and procedures for risk assessment, health and safety checks and the relevant reporting procedures. The trainer should also seek advice from the appointed health and safety person within the organisation if they are unsure but it is advisable to do this anyway in order to clarify procedures and be consistent with any documentation that the organisation uses. If working from home, then the trainer could contact the UK Health and Safety Executive (www.hse.gov.uk) for more advice relating to this area.

If the trainer feels that the organisation's policies could be improved in any way (or there are not any in place), then as a professional in the industry they should discuss this with the health and safety officer within the organisation in order to establish any changes that could reduce the risk of any health and safety issues to either personnel or clients. This is important as the organisation or the trainer could be held responsible for any incidents in which appropriate procedures have not been put in place or implemented.

INJURIES, ILLNESS AND ACCIDENTS

Injuries and accidents are not an uncommon part of personal training sessions. Sometimes clients turn up to sessions when they are suffering from illness, or they suffer a medical emergency during the session as a result of underlying conditions. It's important that trainers become familiarised with their clients enough to identify a drop in performance or a lack of motivation that could be symptomatic with the onset of illness. It is not the role of the trainer to diagnose the illness but it is certainly their responsibility to refer the client to appropriate medical personnel.

DEALING WITH INJURIES

In the cases of a minor injury, treatment may be given on site at the time. If the injury is of a more serious nature, however, then the injured person may require some sort of outside medical attention. It is not possible to list all the possible minor and major injuries but the trainer could use the following list as a guide. For more detailed information relating to minor and major injury treatment, it is recommended to use one of many available first aid books.

- Minor injuries, such as cuts and bruises. These types of injury can be given treatment on site.
- Major injuries include fainting, asthma, overexertion, heat exhaustion, sprains and strains, diabetic emergency, epilepsy and heart failure. These types of injuries require outside medical attention.

Sprains and strains are also known as 'soft-tissue' injuries as they are injuries caused to either muscle, tendon or ligament (soft) tissue. These types of

Table 16.2	RICE procedures	
R	REST	Rest, steady and support the injured part of the body.
I	ICE	Apply an ice pack or cold compress. This will reduce swelling and pain.
C	COMPRESS	Apply gentle compression to help reduce swelling.
E	ELEVATE	Raise the injured part to reduce blood flow to the area.

injuries tend to be the most common in the health and fitness industry. Even though these types of injuries require appropriately qualified people to deal with them (such as physiotherapists) the trainer can still give immediate first-aid treatment to someone with a soft-tissue injury until they can be taken to the relevant specialist for further treatment. The immediate treatment that the trainer can provide for all injuries such as this is known by the acronym RICE. This treatment is done in order to reduce the amount of swelling at the site of the injury. Table 16.2 shows the RICE treatment that can be given.

PROVIDING FIRST-AID

During any activity session it is possible that the trainer may have to deal with a situation that requires immediate treatment or first-aid but may also require the use of the emergency services. It is the responsibility of the trainer to assess the situation and decide on the appropriate action. Every organisation should have their own first-aid policy and reporting procedure that is made available to all trainers. It would be wise for trainers to have a copy of this and to make themselves familiar with it. Trainers should also ensure that they know the whereabouts of the duty first-aider (and how to contact them) at the venue whenever they are

instructing but it is also essential that they hold a current first-aid qualification. Trainers should always make sure that they have information on any client's individual medical background and any injuries, and they should pay particular attention to any allergies that they have been told about. It is also the responsibility of the trainer to make sure that a first aid kit is available at all sessions. This kit should be maintained at all times and should never contain any pills or creams (pills or creams should never be administered by trainers in case of problems such as allergic reactions).

DEALING WITH EMERGENCIES

A trainer may also find themselves in the situation where they have to deal with emergency procedures such as fires, medical emergency, security incidents or missing persons. When dealing with an emergency it is important that the trainer is familiar with the emergency operating procedures (EOPs) that are available from all places of work – if they are not available, then ask for them as they are a legal requirement. The trainer will need to familiarise themselves with the EOP procedures at each site that they work from as they will be different. This will help trainers to make informed judgements as to the requirement of emergency services. As a simple guideline the following procedure can be adhered to during an emergency situation:

1. Assess the situation. Approach quickly but remain calm. Identify any risks to yourself, the casualties and bystanders.
2. If you judge the situation to be life threatening, call the emergency services immediately.
3. Make the area safe. The conditions that caused the emergency may still be a problem and cause even further harm to casualties and others.
4. Give emergency aid. Assess any casualty and give any necessary first aid.
5. Get help. Send someone for help or telephone for assistance.
6. Comfort the casualty. Casualties tend to be in emotional distress. Comfort and reassurance in a calm controlled manner is the best way to support the casualty until help arrives. Reassure the casualty that you are qualified and experienced in these situations.
7. Keep the casualty warm and comfortable.

CONTACTING EMERGENCY SERVICES

When a trainer or a resident first-aider gives emergency aid it is often the case that an emergency service, usually an ambulance, is then required. Sometimes the trainer is a bit reluctant or unsure whether to call the emergency services or not but it is always better to be safe than sorry. You could call them to ask their advice on whether or not they're needed, and they should be able to offer advice.

When calling the emergency services it is important to give the full information and details regarding the nature of the incident and to speak calmly and precisely, describing exactly where the accident has taken place and where on the premises/

grounds you are. If there is a need to call the emergency services, then adhering to the following procedure would be useful:

1. Keep calm and speak clearly.
2. Give your full name and state which service you require.
3. Give the full name, address and telephone number of the club or facility where the session is being held.
4. Give the exact location details and time of the accident/incident.
5. Give the number and condition of any casualties and details of any treatment which is or has been given.
6. Give the access point for the ambulance.
7. Instruct someone to meet the ambulance, which will help them to reach the casualty as quickly as possible.

Before the emergency services arrive, the trainer must deal with the emergency in the correct manner. Any requirement for emergency first aid must be given and any minor injuries dealt with accordingly, otherwise, the casualty must be made as comfortable as possible. All staff at the centre must be informed about the arrival of the emergency services so that clear access can be prepared in advance. As a simple guideline, the following procedure should be adhered to during an emergency situation:

1. Inform the people involved about the correct emergency procedures.
2. Follow procedures in a calm but correct manner.
3. Maintain the safety of those involved at all times.

4. Clearly and accurately report any problems to a responsible colleague.
5. Make a detailed report of the incident afterwards.

According to the Health and Safety (First Aid) Regulations 1981 (www.hse.gov.uk), employers must provide adequate equipment and facilities to enable first aid to be carried out on sick or injured employees. This does not by law extend to customers using the facility, although trainers trained in first aid should make every attempt to administer first aid should the situation arise.

ACCIDENT OR INCIDENT REPORTING

In the event of an accident or an incident occurring during an exercise session in which the trainer is in charge, an accident/incident report must be completed as a record of the event. It is a legal requirement to immediately report all accidents and occurrence of dangerous incidents. The centre from which the trainer is working must provide report forms and procedures for dealing with them. If the trainer is using a public environment for the session, then they must use their own report template to record as much information as possible and then keep this record confidential and safe. As well as being a legal requirement to complete a report, it should also be noted that there is a statutory requirement to keep accident records for a period of at least three years. It is important that an accident/incident report is completed at the earliest available opportunity so that an accurate recall of the event can be made. Should the trainer come across any problems when dealing with an emergency such as fire alarms not working, no first-aid contact or emergency exits blocked they should report this immediately to the relevant person in the facility as well as noting it in the report.

MARKETING IN PRACTICE

THE NOS LEVEL 3 PERSONAL TRAINER CRITERIA COVERED IN THIS CHAPTER ARE:

- Why it is important to plan marketing and sales
- Where you can find out information about your market
- How your market is segmented, for example, by age, income, lifestyle and image, buying habits, occupation and social class, the benefits that potential clients are looking for, etc.
- How to assess the market for your services taking account, for example, of the price of your services, how to promote the service, customer needs and expectations, trends in the industry, etc.
- How to identify your competitors and their strengths and weaknesses
- How to identify your own strengths and weaknesses
- How to develop services that address a certain 'niche' in the market
- How to identify the best ways of reaching your potential clients, for example, by approaching likely clients directly, by using other staff to approach clients on your behalf, by advertising materials, etc.
- The 'image' your clients may have of the types of services you offer and how to develop an image that is unique to you
- How to present your services so that they and their benefits will be attractive to clients
- Different ways you can present your services, for example, by having leaflets printed, by preparing 'scripts' so that you or others can approach clients directly, by commissioning advertisements, by developing website materials
- The importance of being proactive in your marketing – making every effort to reach your potential clients and convincing them of the value and benefits of your services
- The importance of constantly monitoring your marketing and sales activities and outputs and finding ways to overcome problems and improve what you do
- Methods of monitoring marketing and sales

- The importance of having realistic (in terms of the income you need) and achievable targets for your marketing and sales
- How to develop sales and marketing targets
- The importance of being able to evaluate your sales and marketing plans and how to develop ways of monitoring and evaluating marketing and sales
- Why it is important to correctly identify your clients' needs and expectations in relation to the services you offer
- How to identify services that match your clients' needs and expectations
- The relevant documents that need to be completed and why these are important.
- The importance of having as much information, or sources of information, about your services and their benefits available
- How to communicate about your services and their benefits clearly and in a way that will motivate your clients to take them up
- The importance of being accurate in the information you provide – especially in relation to legal requirements covering trade descriptions and sale of goods
- The importance of giving clients the opportunity to ask questions and discuss your services and their benefits

MARKETING

For trainers, marketing is best described as 'the process of communicating the value of a product or service to customers'. Marketing has also been described as the science of identifying appropriate target markets through effective market analysis and market segmentation, as well as understanding consumer buying behaviour and providing superior customer value. The aspects of this particular description will be discussed in more detail later in this section.

Before exploring the area of marketing in relation to the health and fitness environment it would be useful to distinguish between two of the generally accepted classifications of marketing; that of commercial and social.

In general terms the primary aim of commercial marketing is financial (to make a profit and employ staff, for example) whereas in social marketing the primary aim is related to the 'social good' (adopting healthy lifestyles or being made aware of the dangers of smoking for example). In terms of a personal trainer, the type of marketing they need to think about lies somewhere between surviving as a business and providing a service to help improve the health of your clients.

In health and fitness, many of the principles of commercial marketing have been used in social marketing. This was highlighted in early research by Kotler and Zaltman in 1971 when they reported that commercial marketing principles used to sell products to consumers could also be applied to sell ideas, attitudes and behaviours. Examples of this include health promotion campaigns such as the Choosing Health campaign in 2004, and the Health Challenge England campaign in 2006, which were essentially large-scale behaviour-change programmes designed to improve the health of the general public. As early as 1988, the researchers Lefebre and Flora recognised the importance of such campaigns and set out eight essential components related to social marketing. These are:

1. A consumer orientation to realise organisational (social) goals.
2. An emphasis on the voluntary exchanges of goods and services between providers and consumers.
3. Research in audience analysis and segmentation strategies.
4. The use of formative research in product and message design and the pretesting of these materials.
5. An analysis of distribution (or communication) channels.
6. Use of the marketing mix – utilising and blending product, price, place and promotion characteristics in intervention planning and implementation.
7. A process tracking system with both integrative and control functions.
8. A management process that involves problem analysis, planning, implementation and feedback function.

Many social marketing campaigns today follow Lefebre and Flora's model, but trainers working within the health and fitness environment need to adapt some of these components for the commercial market. Even so, it can be seen later in this section that marketing strategies used within the health and fitness environment are clearly based on the components originally suggested by Lefebre and Flora.

THE PT BUSINESS

In the business environment there are many specific terms that may be unfamiliar to the trainer, therefore, for the purpose of this book, terms will be described with the health and fitness environment in mind. A personal trainer's operation can be classed as a business and the services delivered are known as the product. Personal trainers are usually either self-employed or have created a limited company that has a number of employees. The limited company is usually a 'small enterprise' (according to section 248 of the companies Act 1985, a small enterprise has a turnover of less than £2.8 million and less than 50 employees) or a 'micro-business' (as referred to by the Small Business Service 2003) if there are less than ten employees.

The term 'market' simply applies to all potential clients that are available to the trainer whereas 'target market' or 'market segment' refers to a specific or niche group of potential clients who have needs that differ from clients in other parts of the market.

Most trainers in the industry will have a good knowledge of current trends but for those who are contemplating a career as a personal trainer, the Leisure Industry Week convention is possibly a good starting point as this is where both new and established health and fitness concepts are showcased (visit www.liw.co.uk). Another major event in the health and fitness calendar is the annual FitPro convention (visit www.fitpro.com).

One of the key elements to success in any business is that of having a clear marketing strategy from the outset in order to avoid wasted efforts and maximise results. When establishing a marketing strategy, decisions must always be made – where will you work? are you going to specialise in one particular area? is there a section of the community that isn't being catered to that you could target? – but in order to make these decisions, the trainer should systematically collect, analyse and implement marketing information. There are many available models (in terms of stages of marketing within an overall strategy), most, however, are related to larger type businesses, therefore, the trainer could follow a simple format such as the MOVE model as shown in figure 17.1 that has been developed with the health and fitness industry in mind. The MOVE model is a progressive process in that each stage should be completed before moving on to the next stage.

MARKET ANALYSIS

As there are many potential target groups within the health and fitness industry, it is important that the trainer considers each of the groups as potential clients prior to making any decisions in relation to the overall strategy. Identifying specific groups (segmentation as it is better known) is sometimes done by grouping on the basis of certain characteristics such as:

- **Demographic** – age, income, gender, ethnic or educational background.
- **Geographic** – region or postal code.
- **Psychographic** – lifestyle, activities or habits.

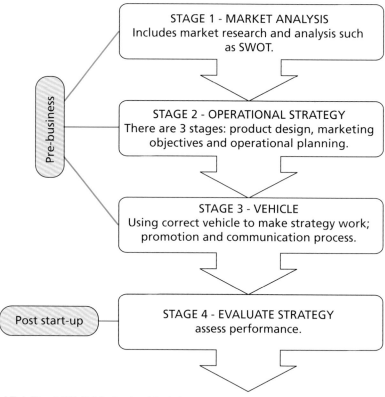

Figure 17.1 The MOVE Marketing Model

- **Behavioural** – how much and how often, brand loyalty.

General trends within these groups can impact the health and fitness market. For example, it has been reported that for the first time in 2007, the number of older adults (of pensionable age) in the UK exceeded the number of under-16-year-olds (Dunell, 2008), a result of people living longer. Also interesting is that the report states that the fastest growing age group is the over-80s. As the number of older adults is forecasted to continue growing, trainers could consider developing initiatives to attract older clients if they had not considered this previously.

Another potential group that the trainer may consider is that of single-person households as according to the Office for National Statistics (ONS 2009a) this number has been growing over the last few decades and now constitutes more than 30% of all households in the UK. There are several sub-groups within single-person households such as those who never marry, and an increasing number of divorcees and widows. Initiatives that include a social aspect, therefore, could be useful in targeting these particular sub-groups.

Standard of living can also have a major impact on lifestyle. Disposable income (how much people have to spend after all deductions) in the UK more than doubled between 1987 and 2006 (ONS, 2008a), however, the country has been in recession since 2008, which will likely have a negative impact on spending. Trainers may well have to adjust their prices to reflect this and also adjust their own lifestyle in order to 'survive' as a business throughout the downturn in the recent economic climate.

In terms of psychographic segmentation, there is overwhelming evidence to show a link between sedentary lifestyles and overweight and/or obesity related problems. Despite significant advances in medicine, the levels of overweight and obesity in the UK continue to be a major concern across all age groups. There have been an increasing number of government initiatives that have been implemented to address the problem which can present an opportunity for trainers to actively seek funding sources to set up programmes that specifically target this particular group.

The groups you target are likely to be a combination of characteristics such as weight loss, older age, rehabilitation, sports and competitors, disability, special populations and group exercise. It is an important decision for any trainer whether to focus on a particular market and develop a reputation as an 'expert' in that field or whether to 'cast the net' as wide as possible in the hope of attracting new clients. If the choice is to focus on a particular group, then it is advised that the trainer gain as many qualifications in the specialist area as possible as being a specialist is often the key to a successful business. Before a decision is made whether to specialise or not, the trainer should carry out research of the market (known as 'market research') in order to gather as much information as possible. To help with this there is access to national survey data via the likes of ACORN, which is a system that classifies neighbourhoods using data from the National Census. Surveys such as the 'Active People' survey in England can identify which activities are most likely to attract paying customers and how participants vary in terms of variables such as income, employment status, socio-economic group and house ownership, etc.

MARKET RESEARCH

Market research can be described as the study of markets (or segments) a business would like to sell a product to. It involves the gathering of data and the conversion of that data into a form that allows the trainer to easily use the information to take appropriate action (the term 'data' simply refers to a piece of relevant information that is useful to the trainer). This data transfer process is sometimes referred to as a 'client management system' and in relation to personal training usually involves the transfer of information from paper format to an appropriate computer software system such as Excel. In terms of market research there are essentially two main types: Primary and Secondary.

Primary research

This relates to the collection of new information to meet the specific needs of the researcher. Methods of collection include 'quantitative' (gathering of numerical information that can be analysed) such as carrying out surveys by phone/post/internet or face-to-face in order to gather information related to specific questions. Take care in wording

Table 17.1	Example of client information areas

Information area	Rationale
Age	Helps to identify age-related groups such as younger or older adults.
Gender	Might help identify specific groups based on gender and also potential for 'buddy systems'.
Income	Helps to build up a general picture of the socio-economic area to help with price pitching.
Occupation	Can help to identify large organisations and sedentary or active lifestyles.
Health conditions	Can help to identify any specialist group such as obesity, diabetes, etc.
Disabilities	Allows appropriate qualifications to be sought.
Hobbies	Helps to identify potential training groups: cycling, jogging, walking, etc.
Current activity level	Builds a picture of the activity levels of potential clients.
Gym membership	Identifies numbers that are currently gym active.
PT trained	Can identify what percentage DO NOT have a PT.
Needs	By identifying the main needs of clients, trainers can specialise.
Barriers	Identifies the main reasons people don't engage with a PT.

MARKETING QUESTIONNAIRE

Dear Sir/Madam

I am in the process of establishing my personal training business in your area and would appreciate your help to make sure that I offer services that are really needed. Please could you take the time to answer the questions below. You are free to withhold any personal information you like but please be assured that all information will be treated confidentially in accordance with the Data Protection Act and will not be shared with anyone else.

Name   Male/female

Address   Post code

Please indicate if you would like me to contact you with further information: ☑ Yes   ☐ No

Age: How old are you?

☐	☐	☐	☑	☐
<16	16–30	31–50	51–65	≥65

Income: Please indicate how much you earn.

☐	☐	☑	☐	☐
<15K	15–25K	25–40K	40–60K	≥60

Occupation: What do you do for work?

☐	☐	☑	☐
Unemployed	Manual	Office	Driving

Other (specify) _____

Health conditions: Do you have any health conditions that you know of?

☐	☐	☐	☐	☐
Obesity	Diabetes	CVD	Asthma	High BP

Other (specify) _____

Disabilities: Do you have any disabilities?

☐	☐	☐	☐	☐
Hearing	Vision	Learning	Speech	Wheelchair

Other (specify) _____

Hobbies: What hobbies do you have at the moment?

☐	☐	☑	☑
Swimming	Jogging	Walking	Cycling

Sport (specify) _____

Current activity level: How many times a week do you do hobbies or exercise?

☐	☑	☐	☐	☐	☐	☐	☐
0	1	2	3	4	5	6	7

Gym membership: Do you regularly attend any gym training?

☑ None ☐ Gym ☐ Aqua ☐ Aerobics ☐ Spinning ☐ Circuits

PT trained: Do you have a personal trainer?

☐ Yes ☑ No

Needs: Are there any health or fitness goals that you would like to achieve?

☐ Weight loss ☐ Fitter ☐ Gain muscle ☑ Stay healthy

Other (specify) _____

Barriers: Is there anything preventing you from exercising regularly?

☐ Cost ☐ Transport ☐ Facilities ☐ Fear ☑ Motivation

Other (specify) _____

Figure 17.2 Example marketing questionnaire (for a template visist: www.bloomsbury.com/9781408187234)

questions – you want to make sure that you get the right type of information. 'Qualitative' methods can also be used which relate to the gathering of descriptive information and would include interview and observation (interviews, however, can be very time-consuming).

Secondary research

This relates to the analysis of information that already has been gathered for another purpose. The advantage of this method is that it is usually faster and less expensive than gathering primary research. Secondary data can be purchased from companies that create databases but the disadvantage is that it often does not contain the specific information that is required.

Whatever method of market research the trainer chooses to identify a potential target market group and their needs, they should carefully consider the type of information that would be useful in terms

of business set-up and progression. Table 17.1 outlines areas of client information that the trainer might find helpful in doing this and a rationale for gathering information in each of the areas.

Having decided on the information areas that are appropriate, trainers need to develop a system of collecting information. This could be a standardised questionnaire or a phone script in order to gather and record the information that makes it easily transferable to the client management system (as with all collected information). Questionnaires are probably the most common market research tool but take care when creating it: a poorly designed questionnaire will generate almost pointless information. Although there are many ways in which to design a questionnaire it is often better to adhere to general guidelines such as the following:

• Keep the questionnaire simple and brief as potential clients can be put off by drawn out or complicated forms.

- Make sure that there are instructions to follow.
- Start with general, easy to complete questions then move to more specific questions that may require some thought process.
- Pre-test the questionnaire and ask for feedback relating to understanding, simplicity and style.
- Tailor the question to the type of response required (scales, rankings, open and closed-ended).

The marketing questionnaire shown in figure 17.2 uses tick box answers for certain questions which is a form of closed-ended question (a question in which the response is limited to a particular choice). Some of the questions allow for a more detailed response, which is known as an open-ended question. These can provide answers that are more useful to the trainer.

Start your questionnaire with a brief introduction stating the purpose and nature of the questionnaire, and make sure that there is a reference to confidentiality. If completing the questionnaire over the phone, this should be one of the first pieces of information that is mentioned. As can be seen in the example in figure 17.2, the person who filled out the questionnaire ticked yes to getting further information. This could prompt the trainer to provide more marketing information relating to the services offered, but also include details on how there are opportunities for training in groups (such as walking or cycling as indicated) or pairing up with a 'training buddy' with a similar profile. This would be done as it was identified that the potential client lacks motivation, would consider a social aspect and is concerned about going to a training situation alone. As the questionnaire also indicates that she is an office worker, information sent out could also state that advice would be given related to fitness at work.

Once information had been sent out to the potential client, the computer management system (such as a diary system in Microsoft Outlook) could be set up to give a prompt (seven days later, for example) to make a follow-up telephone call to the potential client to discuss further. The outcome of the follow-up call could then be recorded on the questionnaire (or on the computer system as preferred).

Once an outcome had been achieved, be it negative or positive, the questionnaire could then be put on file. Depending on the filing system used, this could be placed under headings such as 'rejected', 'contact again' or 'signed up' which are self-explanatory.

Regardless of the outcome, the marketing questionnaire should be used in conjunction with the Enquiry Tracking Form (see page 224) so that a complete record of all client details is made easily accessible. It is useful to store appropriately all marketing questionnaires as they can provide important information in the future, such as that related to market trends. While the trainer is undertaking a form of market research it is also prudent to consider the potential competitors in the area of the proposed business. One of the most common methods of doing this is by using the Strengths Weaknesses Opportunities Threats or SWOT analysis.

SWOT analysis

Knowledge of potential competitors is crucial. It is useful to look at your competitors, how they market themselves and what services they offer, as the analysis can help to identify potential marketing objectives within an overall operational strategy (stage 2 of the MOVE Marketing Model). Regardless of the size of the business, one rela-

STRENGTHS: (What are the strengths of the proposed business compared to those of competitors). For example:
- Can create new image.
- Responsible for own standards.
- Have knowledge of other segments.

WEAKNESSES: (What are the weaknesses of the proposed business compared to those of competitors). For example:
- Not yet established.
- Perception of single operator.
- No experience of delivery.

OPPORTUNITIES: (Usually related to the growth of the business as a result of expansion, diversification or new segment delivery). For example:
- Opportunity to target certain segments that competitors do not deliver to.

THREATS: Mainly related to direct competitors (new entrants, dominance of large operator), indirect competitors (vying for leisure time – cinema's, restaurants). For example:
- Several large operators in area and Business Park with leisure facilities near proposed operating site.

Figure 17.3 Example of a SWOT analysis matrix

tively simple method of doing this is the SWOT analysis as shown in figure 17.3. This method involves focusing on strengths and weaknesses (known as internal factors) and opportunities and threats (known as external factors) that can impact on the proposed business. It should be noted that trainers can only have an effect on internal factors, such as updating their qualifications, whereas they can have little or no effect on external factors.

Although a relatively simple process to implement, trainers would need to devote time to identify potential competitors within the proposed area of operation using sources such as the Internet, newspapers, magazines and direct contact with clubs and other training facilities. Information can sometimes be limited but it is important to try and build up (as best as possible) an overall profile of competitors in order to make comparisons in the SWOT analysis as this can often determine the direction of a new business. This particular process also encourages the trainer to reflect on their own product strengths and weaknesses, which can often

help identify opportunities that otherwise might not have been explored.

OPERATIONAL STRATEGY

Having completed the market analysis stage and collated all relevant information, decisions must be made about the direction of the business, in terms of an operational strategy, in order to gain an advantage over competitors in the marketplace. Typically there are three stages to this particular process: product design, marketing objectives and operational planning.

PRODUCT DESIGN

At this stage the trainer should have an idea of the product that they can offer, and have tailored the product in response to information gathered during the research stage. The concept of design quality is possibly one of the main factors to consider prior to setting marketing objectives. The initial design of the product is crucial as it can create a competitive advantage and aid penetration into the marketplace. The quality of design can also lead to customer loyalty and a willingness to accept. Although there are many facets to design quality, the trainer could focus on three main areas: product levels, brand image and cost.

Product levels

For the purpose of this particular section the product can be thought of in terms of design prior to its delivery (the actual service). When the trainer is in the process of designing the product they should consider what aspects could differentiate the product from its main competitors. This can be done by using the Product Design Pyramid as shown in figure 17.4 which encourages the trainer to consider the product in terms of three levels: core benefits, expected service and augmented product.

- **Core benefits.** From an individual perspective the core benefits of the product should be specific and reflect the client's goals. In wider terms, core benefits would be specific

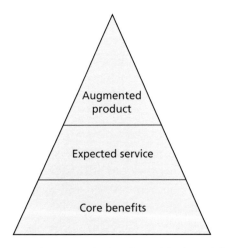

Figure 17.4 Product Design Pyramid adapted from Kotler (1997)

to the chosen target market/s, including areas such as weight loss, performance, health and rehabilitation.

- **Expected service.** This is related to the actual service that the client would expect in order to address the core benefits that had been identified. For example, if weight loss had been identified as a core benefit then the client would expect to receive dietary advice and appropriate aerobic-type exercise sessions. Bear in mind that the perception of the client as to the service they get may well differ from the perception of the trainer, therefore, this should be evaluated on a regular basis.
- **Augmented product.** This is the area that could differentiate the product from those of competitors by offering enhanced features that could improve (or augment) the core benefits and expected service. Once a business started operating, the way in which the service is delivered can often augment the product and make it distinctive above its competitors (often due to word of mouth). During the promotion stage of the business, however, incentives – perhaps the offer of dietary analysis using the latest software application – that improve on the overall product could be used before the business has had a chance to establish a reputation.

Brand image

It is vitally important to stand out from the crowd in a competitive market. One strategy often used to do this is by the creation of a brand image, which can be verbal, visual and psychological in nature. For example, as a starting point, the trainer should consider a business name and logo that has the following attributes:

- Stands out, distinctive, easily recognisable
- Positive in nature
- Memorable
- Can be easily read and pronounced
- Logo reflects the name
- Name and logo relate to the characteristics of the business

In terms of the psychological aspect of the brand image, try to use it to get an initial response but also to develop long-term brand loyalty. Creating an initial response is obviously linked to how well the product is promoted, which is crucial to making potential clients aware of the brand. As potential clients would make assumptions in the early stages based on the image it would be useful for the trainer to consider associations that might help influence their response. For example, a brand that included an affiliation to a professional body such as SkillsActive or REPs or a recognised institute such as the British Heart Foundation would increase the quality perception of the brand. Repeat business should be at the heart of the strategic objectives for all trainers, especially in an ever increasing marketplace where potential customers can be bombarded with choice. Most research in this area relates to high street brands such as Tesco and Boots who encourage repeat business by using incentives such as reward point systems. Trainers could consider the use of similar strategies (albeit on a smaller scale) such as loyalty programmes whereby clients would receive free/

reduced price sessions or assessments in return for long-term financial commitment.

Cost

As with any business, the cost of the product should reflect its value and expected quality but it is a sensitive issue that should be carefully considered as it can ultimately determine the success of any business. Perceived value is a subjective measure, therefore, the trainer should reflect on the design of their individual product levels (core, expected and augmented) as well as information gathered in the market research stage before any pricing decision is made. When trying to determine a product price (in this case an hourly rate is common), it might be useful to think in terms of a 'break-even point' or, in other words, what is the minimum that can be charged per hour in order to cover costs. In order to do this the trainer should make a list of all the costs that would be incurred. It is probably easier to do this on an annual basis, which can then be broken down into monthly or weekly targets. It should be noted at this point that initial start-up costs would obviously be higher, therefore, it would be better to do this for a follow-on year, assuming that the trainer is willing to accept a potentially decreased profit in the first year. A break-even analysis can be done using an example such as that in figure 17.5. As can be seen, some costs will be paid on a weekly or even daily basis whereas others will be paid on a monthly or annual basis (new trainers will need to do some background work in order to estimate potential costs relating to some of the areas). Once all costs have been taken into account, each trainer will need to estimate how many hours per week they are willing to dedicate to face-to-face delivery, bearing in mind that

> **Tip**
> Consider legally registering your logo in order to prevent trademark infringement by competitors.

hours will need to be allocated to administration and also for personal time.

In the example it is assumed that the trainer has set aside a target of twenty hours for face-to-face contact. It is also assumed that realistic costs have been estimated, which have been added together to give a total annual cost (TAC). This total has then been divided by 48 (assuming the trainer has four weeks' holiday each year) to give a total weekly cost (TWC). The TWC can then be divided by the number of hours the trainer expects to deliver to give a final break-even hourly rate. This reflects the minimum amount that the trainer will need to charge with anything above

BREAK-EVEN ANALYSIS

	Weekly	Monthly	Annual
Promotion:			
Advertising (newspaper, magazine, radio)		£120	£1440
Website (including email facility)		£25	£300
Leaflet/flyers			£150
Business cards			£75
Facility:			
Indoor space rental (15hrs)	£150		£7800
Outdoor space rental (5hrs)	£40		£2080
Taster sessions			
Equipment:			
Clothing			£300
Specialist equipment			£500
Travel:			
Petrol	£30		£1560
Public transport	£45		£2340

Total annual cost (TAC)   = £16,545

TAC ÷ 48 = Total weekly cost (TWC)   = £344.68

Break-even point based on 20 hours per week (HPW)   = TWC ÷ 20

         = £344.68 ÷ 20

         = £17.23

Figure 17.5 Example break-even analysis (for a blank template visist: www.bloomsbury.com/9781408187234)

this representing a profit (any profits are subject to taxation, therefore, trainers should familiarise themselves with this area).

MARKETING OBJECTIVES

The clarification of specific marketing objectives at this point would help in the development of an overall operational strategy. An operational strategy can be described as a number of strategies or approaches used to achieve each marketing objective. Most objectives within the PT environment are related to areas such as cost, product and promotion, however, trainers should always be aware that objectives should be designed so that they can be monitored and evaluated (the SMART acronym can help in this process).

S – specific: focus on a specific goal

M – measureable: make the objective quantifiable

A – achievable: make objectives challenging but achievable

R – realistic: objectives must be realistic within the current climate

T – time-based: be specific about the time-frame

PRODUCTS

MARKETS

Protect / build:
• Consolidation
• Market penetration

Product / service development:
• Initial design
• New concept

Market development:
• New segment
• New locations

Diversification:
• Area of delivery

Figure 17.6 Ansoff matrix adapted from Ansoff, H. (1988) Corporate strategy. Penguin, Ch6

Once your objectives have been identified, approaches should be developed in order to achieve the objectives, which form the basis of the operational plan (see figure 17.7). There are several tools that have been designed to help do this including the Ansoff Matrix.

The Ansoff matrix helps the trainer to focus on objectives relating to both the product and the market by addressing the following areas: protect/build, product/service development, market development and diversification.

Protect/build

This part of the matrix encourages the trainer to think about strategies that are concerned with either protecting the current position of the business (for those already in operation) or for building a position (for new businesses). In terms of businesses already in operation, consolidation is considered key to protecting (and strengthening) their position in the marketplace. Trainers should be aware that consolidation does not necessarily mean to carry on as normal as market situations often change due to the actions of competitors, therefore, reshaping and innovation are strategies that can be used to either react to or pre-empt competitors' actions. In terms of new businesses, strategies should be considered that will help to penetrate the existing market. Many factors can affect this, however, competitor complacency and niche markets are often key to market penetration.

Product/service development

When trainers are first entering the market the design of the product should be related to the environment at the time and based on collation of gathered information. However, changes in the environment may create demand for new services,

SWOT ANALYSIS

Strengths	Opportunities	Weaknesses	Threats
Expertise to deliver to specific target market.	Outdoor delivery due to geographical circumstances.	One-person business compared to direct competitors.	Several large H&F clubs in area that provide PT opportunities.

OBJECTIVES:

Protect/build:
- Establish costing plan prior to start-up which considers operational costs.
- Design a management information system and promotional campaign prior to start-up.

Diversification:
- Establish system to regularly assess client demand in terms of diversification.

Market development:
- Develop strategy to identify potential new market segments and promote delivery intention following annual review.
- Establish review system that should include process of sourcing training providers for relevant qualifications and acceptable delivery mode in relation to new segments.
- Include feasibility of staff expansion, geographical expansion in relation to client demands in annual review.

Product/service development:
- Create an inventory of unique selling points prior to promotion campaign.
- Establish three-monthly review to consider new concepts.
- Include feasibility of staff expansion, geographical expansion and client demands in annual review.

ANSOFF STRATEGIES

Consolidation: N/A

Initial design:
Offer pricing plans for long-term commitment. Liaise with university for access to facilities to be able to offer specialist service beyond competitor capability. Identify facility costs to make decision on delivery environment.

Market penetration:
Create website, promo materials, taster sessions and seminars which focus on expertise, cost-plan benefits and environment. Design management information system that addresses all objectives.

New concept:
Subscribe to H&F magazines and attend conferences (LIW, IDEA, etc).

New segment:
Carry out market research to identify demand for new segment and appropriate training. Do cost/benefit analysis for training cost versus potential new segment income. Consider new staff as alternative.

New locations:
Carry out market research to identify potential clients and facilities in wider area.

Area of delivery:
- Survey of client base needs to identify demand for specialist information.
- Do cost/benefit analysis for training cost versus potential specialist delivery income. Consider new staff as alternative.

S ☐   M ☐   A ☐   R ☐   T ☐

Figure 17.7 Example of a micro-business operational plan (for template visist: www.bloomsbury.com/9781408187234)

especially in the health and fitness industry, which has a reputation for 'fad' products. Customers in the industry also tend to be knowledgeable in terms of judging value for money, therefore, trainers should consider the regular introduction of new concepts as a strategic approach.

Market development

When a trainer first starts out they often match their particular expertise and qualifications to a specific segment of the market. If this is too selective, it may limit the trainer's opportunities. If alternative segments are identified during on-going market research, trainers should consider offering their services in order to sustain or develop the business. There is often the need, however, for capability development in that the trainer would need to up-skill in relation to the new segment delivery. The trainer could also choose to target a wider audience in terms of geographical location in order to meet market development objectives. This could involve the trainer travelling to organised group sessions as opposed to clients travelling to the trainer.

Diversification

As well as delivering the service to a range of market segments the trainer could consider diversifying their product into other areas. Many trainers tend to specialise in an area of delivery such as strength and conditioning, biomechanics, psychology and nutrition, however, being able to deliver a quality service in more than one area can at least add value to the service and only help to improve the chances of success.

VEHICLE

Following successful completion of stage 2 (operational strategy) of the MOVE Marketing Model (see page 223), the trainer needs to consider how to deliver essential product information to the potential target market in order to move their business forward. In other words, they need to make appropriate decisions relating to the 'vehicle' that could be used to deliver the information effectively. In order to do this the trainer could focus on three distinct areas that are related to the vehicle: promotion, the communication process and monitoring.

PROMOTION

Once the operational strategy of the business has been completed the trainer needs to promote, by using a variety of techniques, their product's key messages to potential and/or existing clients. In terms of potential clients this should be done using an approach that moves them through the various stages of the 'Purchase Ladder Model', as shown in figure 17.8, which has been adapted from various 'Hierarchy of Effects' models proposed by those such as Sheldon (1902) and Strong (1925). As can be seen, this particular progressive model consists of promoting an awareness of the product, creating or maintaining an interest in the product, then stimulating a desire and hopefully an action to purchase the product (often referred to as 'take-up'.

In the business environment the process of using various promotion methods to achieve the action stage of the Purchase Ladder Model is typically referred to as 'Integrated Marketing Communication' (IMC) which was a concept that was first developed by Delozier in 1978. Over the years much work has been done in relation to the development of the original IMC model. The main reason for this was to try and integrate

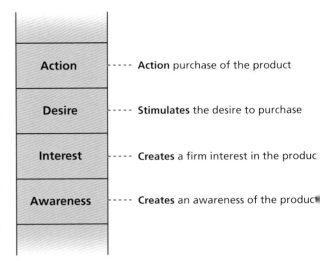

Figure 17.8 Purchase Ladder Model

the more traditional and new communication mediums to effectively provide information to potential consumers. Since then new models, such as the 'promotion mix' or the 'communications mix', suggest that there are many mediums, and components of those, that are effective in doing this. For example, the components of media such as advertising, direct marketing and sales promotions as shown in figure 17.9 (which is adapted

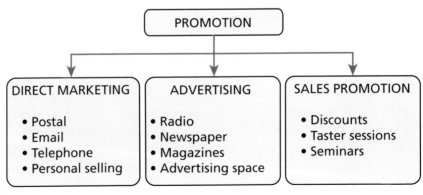

Figure 17.9 Example of promotions mix components

from Blakey, 2011) have all been suggested to be effective promotion tools depending on the individual circumstances of the businesses using them. Depending on the business circumstances there are advantages and disadvantages related to all components as discussed in table 17.2.

Direct marketing

Direct marketing is a tool that can be used for new or existing clients, and be measureable by the way the product is taken up. It can come in many different types, such as postal, email, telephone and personal selling (face-to-face), with each type having advantages and disadvantages as shown in table 17.2. Email promotion tends to be the most frequently chosen format but that is not to say that the postal, telephone and personal selling formats are not without advantages. Postal and email methods tend to be used more when a client base has been established in order to 'drip-feed' information and maintain a good trainer–client relationship, however, telephone marketing is often used in the new business set-up stage as a reactive tool to deal with any incoming enquiries. Personal selling is also a method that tends to be used to generate new clients and is often used in conjunction with sales promotion initiatives (see below).

Advertising

As with direct marketing, advertising is designed to create interest or desire for the product from potential or existing clients. The type of advertising (television, radio, newspapers and magazines, etc.) is determined by how much has been allocated for it in the budget. TV is often seen as too expensive for the trainer, however, as with radio, it is possible to get air time on certain programmes or channels (especially if they are local) if the broadcaster considers that there is benefit to doing so. For example, there are many personal trainers who appear on various TV shows as the resident 'expert', which is invaluable in terms of promotion. Newspapers and magazines can also be a costly option, however, editors are always willing to consider free editorial for certain articles such as trainers having a major impact in the community as a result of delivering 'new' group training sessions.

Sales promotion

Unlike direct marketing, sales promotion is designed to elicit immediate action (final stage of the Purchase Ladder Model) on the part of the potential or existing client by using a time-limited incentive. One of the reasons for using a time limit is to prevent the client from becoming dependent on the incentive, which can impact on the profit of the business. This type of promotion component is a strategy that is often used to increase sales and maintain repeat purchase. Sales promotion techniques can be used as strategies to achieve specific operational objectives. For example, taster sessions can be used as a marketing penetration strategy used to achieve a specific market development objective.

Once trainers have decided which of the promotion components that they intend to adopt, they should then consider the actual process required in which to communicate the key messages of the business. This is simply known as the 'communication process'.

COMMUNICATION PROCESS

As with all strategies, a clear and coordinated approach to the delivery of your message is important as most clients live in a society where they are constantly bombarded with endless messages every day. One way in which to do this is to consider the communication process such as the model in figure 17.10 adapted from Pickton and Broderick in 2004.

Table 17.2	Advantages and disadvantages of promotion mix components	
Promotion component	**Advantages**	**Disadvantages**
Direct marketing: Postal	Can drip-feed subliminal message. Allows personalisation.	• Can be binned before reading. • Junk image. Costly. • Limited format – letters, leaflets, flyers.
Email	Cost effective. Customised. Varied formats – as postal but including DVDs, podcasts, etc.	• Depends on database accuracy. • Can easily unsubscribe.
Telephone	Can answer specific questions.	• Labour intensive.
Personal selling	Personal touch. Can make immediate sign-up.	• Requires personal skills such as listening and empathy. • Labour intensive.
Sales promotion: Discounts	Gets clients to commit to multi-sessions in advance, therefore, creating cash flow.	Can impact on profit margins.
Free taster sessions	Can generate new sales for market expansion or penetration.	Can impact on the amount of hours that are free to deliver to paying clients.
Seminars	Can generate interest to help move to action stage.	Can impact on the amount of hours that are free to deliver to paying clients.
Advertising: Radio	Hits local target market. Low cost.	Audio only so no visual stimulus.
Newspaper/magazines	Widespread coverage. Believability and credibility.	Needs repetition so can be costly. Lengthy process
Advertising space/posters	Constant exposure. Can negotiate cost and location.	Cannot direct at target market.

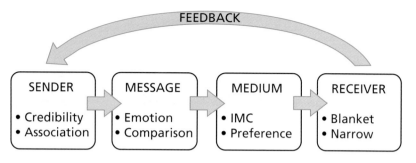

Figure 17.10 The communication process

Sender

The start of the communication process simply relates to the sender of the information, in this case the trainer. Early work by those such as Levitt in 1967 suggests that the trustworthiness of the sender is vital for acceptance of the message by the receiver. For established businesses, there may be a degree of trustworthiness that is attached to the sender by the way they have delivered the product in the past. New businesses are obviously at a disadvantage in this case, however, they could associate themselves with professional organisations (see section on brand image, page 230) in order to establish or increase their initial product credibility perception.

(see pages 230–1)

Note

The Trade Descriptions Act 1968 has been established to prevent service industry providers (PTs fall into this category) from misleading consumers. This law states that companies or individuals who make false claims about the products or services that they sell are committing an offence. Any means of communication relating to the product must be as described, of satisfactory quality, and fit for purpose. For a full explanation visit www.legislation.gov.uk.

Message

Having developed the characteristics of the overall product using the Product Design Pyramid (see pages 230–1) the trainer needs to determine key messages to be communicated to the target market that reflects those characteristics. This is really only limited by the creativity of the trainer, however, key messages in marketing tend to focus on two main areas: emotion and competitor comparison. Messages that relate to emotion could include those that refer to specific health problems and benefits associated with physical activity, whereas messages that relate to comparison might refer to specialist services offered over and above those of competitors. As a way forward, trainers should consider focusing on three main areas in terms of developing the messages to be communicated:

- Make sure there is as much information (or links to sources of information) as possible about the services offered and their benefits so that potential clients can make an informed decision and are not confused about the key messages.

- Create clear and positive messages about the services offered and the related benefits in order to move potential clients towards a positive response.
- Always be accurate in the messages that you communicate as there are legal considerations such as the requirements covering trade descriptions and sale of goods.

Medium

The term medium simply relates to the way in which key messages are then communicated to the target market. Key messages can be communicated via a multitude of media options but this is often down to the preference and expertise of the trainer. Expertise can be bought in at this stage but the cost must be either absorbed or factored into the break-even analysis (see page 232).

Receiver

The communication of key messages, by its very nature, demands the receipt of the sent messages by the receiver. The trainer can choose whether to use a blanket approach by sending the messages to as many potential clients as possible or to use a more specific approach by targeting a more narrowly determined area (target market or segment). In relation to the health and fitness industry, typical segments often targeted by personal trainers include those shown in table 17.3.

Feedback

Regardless of the approach used, feedback from the receiver is essential in order to assess whether or not the key messages the trainer wants to put across have been effective. This supports the early view of Morris and Holman in 1988, who stated that sales people must assess how their source

Table 17.3	Typical personal training target segments
Segment	**Selection**
Health professionals	• General Practitioners (GPs) • Physiotherapists • Osteopaths/chiropractors • Registered dieticians/ nutritionists
Wellness/ beauty	• Beauty therapists • Holistic therapists • Health spas • Hairdressers
Sports clubs	• Team games (football, rugby, cricket, netball, etc) • Running/cycling/triathlon clubs • Swimming clubs
Retail	• Cafes/restaurants • Health food shops • Sports shops (running/cycling, etc) • Clothes shops (especially women's' fashion)
Community	• Schools • Newsagents • Post offices • Community centres

effect is perceived, understood and accepted. There are generally two types of feedback that can give an indication of the effectiveness of the communication.

Firstly, if there is a request for further information, this could indicate either an interest on the part of the receiver which would help move them to the next stage of the Purchase Ladder Model (see page 236) or it could simply highlight a need to improve the original key messages. Secondly, a poor response to the communication could also indicate a need for improvement in the original key messages. Most importantly in terms of feedback, the trainer should always give potential clients the opportunity to ask questions and discuss the services offered and their benefits.

Having considered the communication process the trainer should develop a timeline for the implementation of the chosen promotion components. In other words, the sender delivering the key messages (developed in the operational plan) via appropriate media (selected from the promotion mix) to the receiver (target market) over a specified period of time. A relatively simple and visual way to help do this is by the use of a Gannt chart as shown in figure 17.11. The Gantt chart was originally developed by Henry Gantt in the early 1900s. The chart is actually a type of bar chart that illustrates a schedule that usually incorporates a start and finish date relating to the particular components of a project (in this case promotion components). As can be seen in the example, by using a Gannt chart the trainer has at their disposal a quick visual overview of the promotion component strategy timeline. The chart can be used to indicate how certain strategies can be implemented at specific times throughout the year and can also be used to indicate how certain strategies can be dependent on others. For example, in the weeks leading up to and beyond the Christmas period there are opportunities to target those who might want lose weight after bingeing during the holiday period, therefore, a blanket approach might be appropriate for the trainer to use at this time.

The chart can also indicate how certain strategies can be dependent on others, for example, follow-up emails and telephone calls to potential clients might be appropriate in the period just after they have received postal information (this can be seen by the use of red in the relevant boxes). Once a timeline for the promotion components has been designed it is important to be able to

PROMOTION COMPONENT GANNT CHART												
COMPONENT												
Postal	▓			▓			▓			▓		
Email		▓			▓			▓			▓	
Telephone		▓			▓			▓			▓	
Discount												
Tasters												
Seminars												
Radio												
Magazines												
	Jan	Feb	Mar	Apr	May	Jun	July	Aug	Sep	Oct	Nov	Dec

Figure 17.11 Typical Gannt chart

track each component being used by implementing a monitoring system.

MONITORING

Tracking or monitoring is an essential activity as it can help to evaluate the effectiveness of each promotion component, both at the implementation stage of the business and on an on-going basis. Depending on the type of promotion component used, the measure of effectiveness will be different. This measure is often referred to as a 'key performance indicator' or KPI (see figure 17.12). For example:

- **Postal:** if the trainer has decided to target various regional areas based on segmentation characteristics such as geographical or socio-economic, codes could be added to the various promotional materials so that when there is an enquiry from a potential client, the code could be requested. This can help the trainer to identify which areas have the best response rate.
- **Email:** this can be done in a variety of ways. For example, in the early stages of generating interest, websites can be designed to track the number of 'hits' which can then be compared against the number of email enquiries generated from those hits (known as an enquiry to hits ratio). Another way of monitoring an email system is to compare the number of responses to the number of direct emails sent (response to send ratio). Outcomes can then be calculated in percentage terms.
- **Telephone:** if a cold-calling strategy is used, then a simple monitoring method would be to compare the interest shown (request for more information or an initial meeting) against the number of calls made which can then be

calculated as a ratio. If the call was made in response to a query, then the trainer must ask the potential client what it was that generated that initial interest.

- **Taster and seminar sessions:** it can be assumed that those attending seminars and taster sessions already have an interest in the product, therefore, the progression to take-up (action stage of the Purchase Ladder Model) should be higher with this type of promotion. The number of those who take up the product can be compared to the number attending the session and calculated as a ratio.
- **Radio and magazines:** as strategies that are often used to generate interest, potential clients could be asked (via the medium) to quote the particular source when responding either by telephone or email. This can then be monitored as an overall number of responses to a particular time-frame of either radio or magazine advertisements.

In the example shown in figure 17.12 it can be seen that for each individual promotion component, actual KPI outcomes can be compared to targets set in order to give an outcome that would either meet, be above or be below those set targets. Once a business has been established for a considerable period of time, the targets that are set could be established based on results from previous periods.

The example shows that the outcome of several components were above the targets set, which indicate that the strategies associated with each component resulted in favourable responses for that particular time period. Whenever outcomes have been calculated it becomes the decision of the trainer to choose which strategies to continue with. Comparing the cost of each strategy to the

Period: Jan 20XX to: Dec 20XX

Component	KPI	Target	Actual	Outcome	Flag
Postal	Area codes:	A – 120	A – 114	-6	▼
		B – 100	B – 123	+23	▲
		C – 100	C – 102	+2	▲
Email	Enquiry to hits ratio:	1 to 50	1 to 40	+20%	▲
Telephone	Interest to calls ratio:	1 to 50	1 to 70	-40%	▼
Tasters	Take-up to attendance ratio:	1 to 3	1 to 3	0	▶
Seminars	Take-up to attendance ratio:	1 to 5	1 to 4	+20%	▲
Radio	Response rate:	150	125	-25	▼
Magazines	Response rate	200	340	+140	▲

KEY: ▼= below target ▶= on target ▲= above target

Figure 17.12 Example KPI monitoring form (for a template visist: www.bloomsbury.com/9781408187234)

outcome in order to identify its cost effectiveness can help to inform the decision.

It can also be seen in the example that the outcome for some of the components was below the target set which requires consideration on the part of the trainer in relation to each component. It could be that the responses were influenced by a particular time period and, therefore, the trainer might choose to persist with the strategy or the trainer may choose to re-evaluate the target but accept the associated strategy. Whatever monitoring method the trainer uses it should be carried out on a regular basis. The trainer will also need to develop a system in which to monitor enquiries from potential clients in order to provide them with the most effective response to progress them to the take-up stage. The use of a simple enquiry tracking form can be used, such as the example shown in figure 17.13.

In terms of tracking enquiry details, the enquiry tracking form should be used in conjunction with the marketing questionnaire as discussed on pages 226–7. The tracking form is self-explanatory in that when an initial enquiry is made by a potential client, the trainer records specific details such as how the individual first heard of the product. In the example it can be seen that an enquiry was made following receipt of a third postal leaflet. This is useful to record as it gives an indication of the success of the particular promotion component strategy used and also the number of times it was used before a response was initiated.

Once all the potential client details have been recorded the trainer can decide on an appropriate response, which should also be recorded (make sure that dates of the initial enquiry and any responses are included). Depending on the success of the response, the form allows for an outcome to the response to be recorded. The outcome may require the trainer to action another response or it could stimulate the potential client to move to the final take-up stage of the Purchase Ladder Model. The particular stage of the enquiry can be recorded at the foot of the form and filed appropriately so that the trainer is aware of any actions and timelines in which they are required.

EVALUATE STRATEGY

Once the first three stages of the MOVE Marketing Model have been completed, it can be assumed that the business has been operating for a while before the implementation of the final stage: evaluate strategy. As with all successful businesses, regular evaluation is key in order to make timely

---

ENQUIRY TRACKING FORM

Name. Jane Smith   Dob: 25.12.19XX   ~~Male~~/female

Address: 21 Mount Pleasant Drive, Midsummer.   Post code: XX12 6XX

Component	Enquiry detail	Date	Response	Outcome
Postal	Area code: X333 Occurrence: 3rd leaflet	19/8/23	Invited to taster session on 28/8/23.	
Email	Occurrence:			
Telephone	Occurrence:			
Tasters	Which:			
Seminars	Which:			
Radio	Which:			
Magazines	Which:			
Word of mouth	By whom:			

STATUS: ☑ Enquiry stage   ❏ Firm interest   ❏ Signed up

Figure 17.13 Example enquiry tracking form (for a template visist: www.bloomsbury.com/9781408187234)

SERVICE QUALITY QUESTIONNAIRE

Client name   Date

Please read the questions below and circle how satisfied you feel on a scale of 1–10 (10 being the best).

Customer needs: How satisfied do you feel that the service meets your needs in relation to your goals?

☐ ☐ ☐ ☐ ☐ ☐ ☐ ☐ ☐ ☐
1 2 3 4 5 6 7 8 9 10

Cost: Do you feel that the service is good value for money?

☐ ☐ ☐ ☐ ☐ ☐ ☐ ☐ ☐ ☐
1 2 3 4 5 6 7 8 9 10

Convenience: Does the service seem convenient from the perspective of timing?

☐ ☐ ☐ ☐ ☐ ☐ ☐ ☐ ☐ ☐
1 2 3 4 5 6 7 8 9 10

Communication: Do you feel that you are given enough regular information that you can understand?

☐ ☐ ☐ ☐ ☐ ☐ ☐ ☐ ☐ ☐
1 2 3 4 5 6 7 8 9 10

Confidence: Do you feel confident about the knowledge and expertise of the trainer?

☐ ☐ ☐ ☐ ☐ ☐ ☐ ☐ ☐ ☐
1 2 3 4 5 6 7 8 9 10

Context: Are you happy with where the sessions take place?

☐ ☐ ☐ ☐ ☐ ☐ ☐ ☐ ☐ ☐
1 2 3 4 5 6 7 8 9 10

Conducting: Are you happy with the way the service is delivered?

☐ ☐ ☐ ☐ ☐ ☐ ☐ ☐ ☐ ☐
1 2 3 4 5 6 7 8 9 10

Do you have any other comments you would like to make related to satisfaction:

Figure 17.14 The 7Cs Service Quality Questionnaire (for a template visist: www.bloomsbury.com/9781408187234)

and appropriate changes. One of the main ways in which to assess the success of the overall marketing strategy is to evaluate the quality of the service.

SERVICE QUALITY

The quality of the service (like the design) is totally subjective as each potential customer may view the same service differently. However, as perception of service relates directly to the satisfaction of expectations, it is crucial that trainers promote only that which they are confident can be delivered. One of the main problems associated with this is how to assess service quality. In other words, how does the trainer assess how their service meets the needs and expectations of clients? This is an important process as each client

The 'C'	Quality gap	Strategy
Customer needs	Understanding	Carry out market research by adapting the marketing questionnaire (see pages 226–7) to suit in order to reassess customer needs and potential market segment. Develop consultation skills such as listening and empathy.
Cost	Pricing level	Carry out further SWOT analysis (see page 229) of competitors as pricing structures may have changed. Consider sales promotion strategies such as discounts and taster sessions. Link offers to attainment of goals.
Convenience	Locality and time	Consider new marketing development strategies. Are your premises local and accessible? Is there parking or bus routes? Can you be mobile and do home visits? Can the timing of the session be changed to suit the client's schedule?
Communication	Communication	Identify if information is pitched at the correct level or if there is a lack of communication strategy. Re-visit communication methods by considering components from the promotion mix (see page 236). Word of mouth is great but your marketing materials need to reflect the strengths of your product such as your expertise, your ability to achieve results, etc.
Confidence	People	Identify the aspects to be improved such as communication, setting, professionalism, knowledge base, empathy, pushy, hard sell, etc. All aspects can impact on client confidence but revisit the product levels within the Product Design Pyramid (see page 230).
Context	Physical environment	Clients are paying money, therefore, have expectations relating to the training environment. Is it an environment the client will feel comfortable in? Re-think the environment in which the sessions take place. Speak to hotels, clubs, universities, local authorities in relation to use of facilities.
Conducting	Conducting the process	The way you conduct yourself and your sessions is crucial for client adherence. Using a systemised approach can give consistency and demonstrate professionalism. Make sure your systems are in place before you start your business.

Figure 17.15 Example of strategies in relation to identified quality gaps

may identify a different element of the service as their primary satisfaction component. Clients often subconsciously estimate how satisfied they feel from their comparison of what they expected to receive with what they perceived they received. Even the very nature of getting trainers to think about their service should be effective in creating a better service, however, it is best to use a systematic approach rather than relying on self-perception. The 7Cs Service Quality Questionnaire as shown in figure 17.14 can be used for this purpose.

In using the questionnaire, clients are asked to rate their satisfaction (on a scale of 1–10) for each of the 7Cs. A score deemed low by the trainer (this should be set by the trainer) would indicate that the service did not meet the needs of the client (this is otherwise known as a 'quality gap'). Depending on the outcome of the completed questionnaire, the trainer could focus on strategies to improve the identified quality gaps as in the example in figure 17.15.

SELLING
// IN PRACTICE

18

THE NOS LEVEL 3 PERSONAL TRAINER CRITERIA COVERED IN THIS CHAPTER ARE:

- The importance of being proactive in selling without giving the impression of 'the hard sell' and how to do so
- The types of buying signals that a client might give that will help you to move the sale on and how to use these
- The importance of being able to negotiate services that meet the client's needs and your own and how to negotiate a sale
- How to confirm the client is ready to complete the sale without making them feel rushed and why this is an important stage
- Why it is important to agree terms with the client and how to do so

SELLING

Even though marketing and sales are distinctly different it is clear that they have the same goal: marketing is concerned with processes, systems and strategies whereas sales is concerned with accomplishing what marketing proposes. In other words, marketing can greatly influence sales by improving the selling environment. Authors such as Donaldson (1993) promote the concept that selling is a vital part of successful marketing plans. Indeed the role of selling is imbedded in the components of the marketing promotional mix (see page 236). For the self-employed trainer there will be a dual role of developing the marketing strategy and employing promotional techniques identified within it. Selling ultimately involves the identification of a sales opportunity (using strategies identified in the marketing operational plan) and the conversion of that opportunity into a sale. If the needs of potential clients have been correctly identified and interpreted, then matching the service to those needs can improve the chances of sales success. There have been many theories of selling proposed over the years but the trainer should be aware that models or processes based on these theories should be flexible as selling often depends upon circumstances. Some of the most common theories and processes are shown in table 18.1.

As mentioned in table 18.1, some of the first selling theories and processes date back to the early 1900s. Over the years, many have been adapted to suit particular environments, however, similar characteristics have emerged (and been maintained). Adapted from various models, figure 18.1 shows a typical selling process based on several common characteristics. As marketing and sales are inextricably linked it is evident that the first five stages of the selling process relate to marketing theory whereas the last stage of the selling process is within selling theory.

Stage 1: Prospecting

In sales terms this is related to the search for customers, the laborious 'leg work' that is done at the start of the business set-up. In marketing terms this relates to market research and can be achieved by the use of the marketing questionnaire (see pages 226–7) to gather data, which can help to identify potential clients within a target area.

Stage 2: Qualifying

This particular stage is known for identifying 'prospects' from 'suspects'. A suspect is the sales term for someone who has not displayed an interest in the product whereas a prospect has. In marketing terms this relates to the identification of a target market or segment using the data gathered from market research.

Table 18.1	Common selling theories and processes
Theory or process	**Description**
Stimulus-response (or classical conditioning).	Early work by Pavlov (1927) led to much research in the area of trying to condition a response to a particular stimulus. In sales, this would represent key messages designed to stimulate a buyer's needs or desires.
The AIDR model (variations include AIDAS and AIDA).	The attention, interest, desire and resolve model proposed by Sheldon in 1902 is a much debated approach that promotes the idea of sequential steps taken during a selling process. As with all models such as this they need to be flexible in order to identify customer needs and present solutions.
Needs-satisfaction (need, solution, purchase, satisfaction).	Further work by Strong in 1925 that took the behaviour into account which previous models had not.
Buyer-seller similarity.	Research in a variety of environments has often found that the greater the similarity between the seller and the buyer the greater will be the salesman's influence.

	Stage	**Marketing link**
Marketing theory based	Stage 1 – prospecting	Market research (marketing questionnaire)
	Stage 2 – qualifying	Analysis of marketing questionnaire
	Stage 3 – identifying need	Prospect enquiry (tracking form)
	Stage 4 – identifying solutions	Analysis of tracking form for solutions
	Stage 5 – presenting	Solution delivery (from promotion mix)
Selling theory based	Stage 6 – closing	

Figure 18.1 The selling process and marketing links

Stage 3: Identifying need

In sales terms this is the stage at which the first direct contact with the prospect occurs in order to identify a need for the product. In marketing terms this would be related to a prospect enquiry that was made as a result of a promotional strategy, which was then monitored using the enquiry tracking form (see figure 17.13).

Step 4: Identifying solutions

Depending on the nature of the enquiry, it is often the case that prospects require further information in relation to the product or the service. At this stage the trainer would need to identify what information would best suit each individual prospect and record this using the enquiry tracking form.

Stage 5: Presenting

Once the trainer has identified the relevant information that is needed by a prospect it would then be necessary to present this information in a format that would be considered most effective. Formats might include those from the promotion mix (see table 17.2).

Stage 6: Closing (take-up)

This is the stage at which the opportunity is converted into a sale and requires specific skills on the part of the trainer, for example, the ability to ask 'closing' questions and recognise 'buying signals', such as when a prospect asks questions related to details that will occur after take-up or trying to negotiate a better deal.

It is evident that the trainer should arrive at stage six having completed all the stages of the Move Marketing Model (see page 223) including the development of an operational plan. Once at the closing stage of a potential opportunity the trainer needs to be aware of common barriers to selling and how to use strategies to facilitate them.

BARRIERS AND FACILITATORS TO SELLING

Much research has been done in the area of barriers and facilitators to selling, however, common themes appear regardless of the context or the market classification. Those considered useful to the environment of the trainer can be seen in table 18.2.

It can be seen that barriers to selling are very much linked to the area of behavioural change as discussed in chapter 3. Trainers should re-visit some of the strategies related to uptake of exercise as they may be appropriate at the closing stage of the selling process. Overcoming barriers in order to complete the sale often requires a range of abilities on the part of the trainer which are otherwise known as 'seller attributes'.

SELLER ATTRIBUTES

Although there are many books on the subject, there is no such thing as the ideal sales person. All selling situations are unique and should be adapted for each situation, therefore, a good salesperson ought to be adaptable and flexible in order to meet the demands of their customers. Here are some other attributes that a good salesperson should have:

Enthusiasm

Most research agrees that sellers must be enthusiastic about their product and themselves. Early research by Bettger in 1949 paved the way for a vast amount of studies that suggest that this was one of the main characteristics that turned

| Table 18.2 | Barriers and facilitators to selling |

Barrier	Facilitator
Fear of change: People are often reluctant to change which can be affected by the lack of education relating to the product or service.	At this particular time the negatives outweigh the positives, therefore, the trainer needs to consider ways in which to focus on and accentuate the positive aspects of the product (see pre-contemplation stage of behavioural change).
Inertia: Even though people might be willing to change they often don't unless they perceive a better product.	This relates to the quality of the product. If the prospect perceives the product as having quality, they are much more likely to change.
Fear: People often have a reluctance to change based on fear of failure and fear of the unknown.	Word of mouth is an effective tool in allaying the fears of potential clients. Use testimonials from previous clients and employ strategies such as buddy or group training.
Timing: As the behavioural change model alludes to, the timing of change is crucial.	It may be that prospects are not at the right stage of the change model. Re-think the timing strategy and re-visit when appropriate.

failure into success in selling. Enthusiasm is a difficult concept to describe let alone measure yet has been linked to hard-working people and perseverance.

Persuasiveness

Potential clients are faced with an abundance of choice in a competitive market, therefore, the trainer needs to persuade prospects that the product will be of benefit to them. Identifying their needs and matching the product to them is an essential part of this process.

Empathy

This refers to the ability to feel as others. Trainers must be able to listen to prospective clients in order to identify what their needs are and be able to overcome any problems in a way in which the client perceives as understanding. This would require good listening skills on the part of the trainer.

Sincerity

This is a very-much-respected quality in anyone, not just a seller. If a trainer has belief in the value and honesty of their product, then this will easily be portrayed in their manner. People can be reticent when not given the entire facts, therefore, it is always recommended to give as much factual detail as possible and avoid any omissions or evasions when dealing with questions.

Communication

People often make judgements based on verbal communication within the first few seconds, therefore, it is essential to make a good first impression. Trainers could consider the use of the four Ps when in a selling situation.

- **Pace.** People tend to talk at about 140 words per minute. This is fine when talking enthusiastically about a general point but try to slow down to about 100 words a minute when delivering important information.
- **Pitch.** There is nothing more effective in losing a person's interest than a monotone voice. Try modulating the tone of your voice up and down to accentuate certain points.
- **Pronounce.** Having an accent is absolutely fine but try not to use slang words and try to pronounce all words clearly.
- **Project.** In situations such as group presentations or seminars be sure to increase the level of your voice. Project your voice just over the tops of the audience's heads.

One of the most effective forms of communication when selling face-to-face is that of body language. Research in this area generally shows that almost 90% of the effectiveness of communication is attributable to non-verbal methods (see page 80). This includes making eye contact and using positive gestures. Trainers should also look for body language clues on the part of the prospect such as folded arms, which indicates reluctance or leaning forward and nodding, which indicates an expression of interest. There are many training courses available to the trainer that deal in the area of body language such as those on Neuro-linguistic Programming (NLP).

Determination

As in any industry, the trainer will receive more 'no' responses than 'yes' responses. Trainers must show a degree of patience when this is the case but must also be persistent in their approach as potential clients often don't say yes in the first instance.

There is often a mismatch between the needs of the buyer and the aims of the seller, therefore, a determined trainer is one who responds to this as a positive challenge rather than seeing the challenge as insurmountable.

THE CLOSING SALE

For many trainers, the final stage of the selling process (known as closing) is often the stage that they find the most difficult, and often comes with experience. It helps if the trainer is able to recognise buying signals so that at that point they can let the sale happen as a matter of course. As mentioned previously, buying signals include when a prospect asks questions related to details that will occur after take-up or when they try to negotiate a better deal than the one offered. If a trainer has recognised an interest from a prospect, they could try to move towards a firm sales commitment. The use of 'closing' questions at this point is a useful strategy to employ. Closing questions would include those such as:

- What would be a good starting date for you?
- Would you prefer a block-booking rather than session-to-session?
- When would you like to attend a taster session?
- Would you like to take advantage of the current promotion?
- Are you ready to commit to a programme of exercise?
- Would you like to train with a 'buddy' when we start?

It is important at this point to get a firm commitment without appearing be pushy, otherwise the prospect may sense they are being pushed into a sale. One way to move forward at this point is to invite the prospect to a face-to-face meeting on the premise that there will be a negotiation of the services to best meet the prospect's needs. Meeting the prospect face-to-face is a crucial step as this is where negotiation takes place and relevant 'take-up' documents can be completed.

One of the most important documents is the 'service agreement' between the trainer and client as it can help to protect the trainer from liability. When designing a service agreement trainers have several options. They can either enlist the help of a legal firm to help compile the agreement or they can design the agreement themselves and have a legal firm check the final document. Alternatively, they might choose to design the agreement themselves and not enlist the help of a legal firm. If this is the case, there are several areas of information that would be considered important to include.

Medical history

A section should be included to state that screening has taken place (using appropriate methods) and all pertinent medical history has been disclosed and dealt with appropriately depending on the outcome of the screening.

Release of liability

The agreement should act as what is known as a 'waiver of liability' and should be signed by the trainer and the client and a copy retained by each. This is essentially a legal document to state that a person who participates in an activity has acknowledged the risks involved in his or her participation.

Risk awareness

Agreements should acknowledge risks associated with exercise, and by signing the contract the

PERSONAL TRAINING SERVICE AGREEMENT

Name:

Address:

Home Phone: Work/Other Phone:

Emergency contact name: Number:

Trainer's Responsibilities:

1   The trainer will design a personalised programme of exercise based on the client's needs and goals.

2   Each session is typically 45 minutes to 1 hour long.

3   The trainer will provide guidance regarding proper exercise techniques.

4   The trainer will maintain a record of client progress and provide necessary feedback.

5   The trainer will provide on-going evaluation and modification of the programme as necessary according to the client's progress, needs, and goals.

6   If the trainer is late for any session, that time is owed to the client.

7   The trainer will endeavour to notify the client four hours prior to a session if they intend to cancel.

8   All information relating to the client is confidential and will be treated in accordance with the Data Protection Act.

Client's Responsibilities:

1   For sessions on an on-going basis, payment must be received prior to the session. For block bookings, full payment must be made 7 days prior to the start of the first session.

2   Client is expected to discuss all health history information and any medical concerns with the trainer.

3   Client lateness is considered part of the session and is non-refundable (family emergencies or sudden illness will be exempt).

4   The client must give four hours notice for session cancellation. Failure to do so will result in forfeiture of one session (family emergencies or sudden illness will be exempt).

5   The client will communicate any discomforts, pain or concerns experienced during or arising from a session.

6   If the client, for any reason, does not use all of their sessions in the block booking, no refund will be given.

In consideration of participation in a Personal Training Programme, I understand that I must purchase a single session or package of training sessions (block booking) and must read, agree to and sign this agreement.

I understand that the programme designed by the trainer is voluntary and I may be required to undergo a health and fitness assessment that will be fully explained to me. I agree to complete the medical history questionnaire/s accurately and completely including disclosure of any prescribed medications I am taking and any exercise or diet limitations I am aware of or have been informed of by my doctor and any changes that may occur.

I understand that I have the right to stop at any time during a session and that I should inform the trainer immediately of any symptoms such as fatigue, shortness of breath or chest discomfort.

I understand that exercise involves certain risks, including but not limited to, spinal injuries, heart attack, stroke, death and injuries to bones, joints or muscles, however, I agree to voluntarily participation in the exercise programme and assume all risks.

I declare that I have read, understand and agree to the contents of this agreement in its entirety. I do hereby waive, release and discharge the trainer from any and all claims or liability for any present and future injuries or damages resulting or arising from my participation in any activities including but not limited to exercise, personal training or use of the equipment including any injuries and damages caused by the negligent act or omission of any of those persons or entities mentioned above.

Client signature:

Printed Name: Dated:

Trainer signature:

Printed Name: Dated:

Figure 18.2 Example of a service agreement (for a template visit: www.bloomsbury.com/9781408187234).

client assumes all risks pertaining to the training and releases you of liability for any resulting injury or illness.

Consent to testing

The agreement should inform the client about potential health/fitness tests that may take place. Information relating to the tests could be given on a separate document prior to the tests taking place.

Payment

Agreements should always state in detail how much each training session or group of discounted sessions will cost, as well as when payment is expected. It should also state details about consequences for client lateness and cancellations as well as conditions for refunds.

Contact Information

It is important to make sure that the agreement

includes contact information for both the trainer and the client (and also an emergency contact for the client) and this is updated if there are any changes.

Responsibilities

It is useful to include a section that outlines the responsibilities of both the trainer and the client so that everything is fully explained up front and there are no hidden 'surprises' or misunderstandings.

As can be seen in the example service agreement in figure 19.2, details of both the client and an emergency contact have been included; hopefully the emergency contact may never be needed, but in the event of an illness or emergency this might be necessary. It is then useful to outline the responsibilities of both the client and the trainer. The more detail included in this section the better informed the client will be.

The next section contains all the information relating to a 'waiver of liability' and outlines risks associated with exercise. This is the section for which trainers could enlist the help of a legal firm if they feel the need to do so.

Finally, two agreements need to be signed by both the client and the trainer and a copy kept by each. As always, copies kept by the trainer should be done so in accordance with the Data Protection Act.

PRACTICAL FINANCIAL MANAGEMENT

19

THE NOS LEVEL 3 PERSONAL TRAINER CRITERIA COVERED IN THIS CHAPTER ARE:

- How to cost your services and develop marketing and sales plans that take account of cash flow and tax considerations
- The importance of testing your proposed products and services with other people and how to do so

Financial management can be thought of as the process of monitoring, evaluating and controlling the income and expenditure of a business which would include areas such as accounting, reporting and budgeting. Most management systems are more suited to limited companies, however, an understanding of the systems can always benefit the self-employed trainer.

The first stage in the development of a financial management system is to decide whether or not to outsource some or all of these services. If the trainer decides to manage certain areas then there are several software packages available for services such as bookkeeping and accounting. Bookkeeping simply refers to the daily management of the business in terms of recording all transactions that take place. An accounting system, however, is the bigger picture of how the business runs and is the system in place that is responsible for record-

Note

Her Majesty's Revenue and Customs (HMRC) is the authority that requires specific information relating to the profits or losses of a business so that they can calculate any tax payments or refunds as necessary. Whether the intention is to become self-employed or a limited company, there are several areas of financial management that trainers should familiarise themselves with such as budgeting, income statements and cash-flow forecasts.

ing and communicating financial information about the business. If a trainer is self-employed, the only financial information that needs to be communicated is a tax return that is sent annually to HMRC (and is self-explanatory). For limited companies, however, detailed financial reports are required. In this case the trainer can choose to manage the financial system up to a certain point before a qualified Chartered Accountant prepares reports prior to submission to appropriate government agencies.

BUDGETING

Deciding on the allocation of funds to various parts of the business is known as 'budgeting', which is essentially a plan of action expressed in financial terms. Major decisions in any business include deciding how much to invest and the beginning and what percentage of sales to allocate to marketing. In the case of the latter this usually accounts for about 2% of gross sales once the business is established with a higher percentage allocated in the early stages.

Those new to budget planning may find it a difficult process, however, it can often raise concerns that might not have been previously identified such as are the sales targets realistic or can the start-up budget cover the costs of the marketing strategy? On the other hand, a budget plan done realistically can help to decide the feasibility of strategies such as additional staff, expansion, diversification and sales campaigns.

Once trainers become familiar with budget planning it can often help to avoid potential future financial problems. A good place to start the budgeting process is to consider the categories of potential expenditure over the course of the first year and project the costs involved which will be made up of variable expenses such as equipment purchases and advertising, and fixed expenses such as facility rental. Once the total budget costs have been forecasted the trainer could then calculate how many hours they would need to deliver

in order to make a profit at a price that was realistic in terms of the current marketplace (this is a simple method that should be used for feasibility only prior to start-up).

Example:
- Annual budget forecast = £10,500 therefore, break-even requires:
- 420 sessions at £25 per hour = approx 1 session per day or
- 210 sessions at £50 per hour = approx 1 session every other day

Once a business is established, however, forecasting income and expenditure becomes easier as the previous year's information can be used as a basis on which to make budgeting decisions. A system that is often used to provide such information is known as an income statement.

INCOME STATEMENT

Also known as a 'profit and loss (P&L) statement', an income statement simply shows income and expenditure for a given time period.

Once a business is in operation the income statement produced for a completed period can show the profit or loss in relation to that period. Essentially the statement should show all sources of income (or turnover) and all sources of expenditure. The total expenditure is then subtracted from the total income, which gives the profit or loss related to that particular time period. The example in figure 19.1 shows some of the common elements of an income statement related to a personal training business. It can be seen in the example that income from gross sales relates

INCOME STATEMENT

Company: PTs R US

Income Statement period 1 January 2013 to 31 December 2013

INCOME

Gross Sales	36,400	
Less returns and allowances	1,000	
Net Sales		35,400

COST OF GOODS

Purchases (equipment)	4,000	
Cost of Goods Sold		4,000
GROSS PROFIT		31,400
Interest Income	500	
Total Income		31,900

EXPENSES

Salaries	6,500	
Rent	2,300	
Office Supplies	200	
Insurance	100	
Advertising	650	
Telephone	300	
Travel	500	
Total Expenses		10,550
Net Income		21,350

Figure 19.1 Example Income Statement (for a template visit: www.bloomsbury.com/9781408187234)

to the number of sessions that the trainer predicts or actually delivers. Also, an income statement usually contains a 'less returns and allowances', which in this case would relate to circumstances where clients had paid up front for a particular number of sessions but refunds may have been given (based on goodwill) due to unavoidable non-attendance. When this amount is subtracted from the gross sales it is termed the net sales. The cost of goods in relation to the personal training environment is usually as a result of equipment purchases that the trainer requires for delivery of the sessions. When this amount is subtracted from the net sales it is usually termed the 'profit from sales' (or margin). Any banking interest added to this amount is known as the gross profit. All expenses that the trainer incurs must then be subtracted from the gross profit in order to give the final 'net income'.

In terms of budget forecasting for a forthcoming year, this could be done on the basis of comparing the previous year's budget to the completed income statement. For example, a template could be set up to compare the information from the income statement (see figure 19.2) to the budget forecast in order to identify any variances and make subsequent adaptations. As can be seen in the example, a flag (indicated by the tick) could be raised to indicate where the variance was substantial enough to warrant attention from the trainer in terms of adjustment to the budget forecast or adaptation of strategies related to that particular category.

Another method of analysing the cash income and expenditure during a particular time period is by using a 'cash flow statement', otherwise known as a forecast (see figure 19.5).

CASH FLOW STATEMENT (CFS)

It may sound obvious, but in terms of the success of a business, more money needs to be coming in than going out. This is known as cash flow management and enables a business to predict peaks and troughs in cash balance. This can help in terms of planning for contingencies and many banks require cash flow forecasts before considering a loan. Although similar in many ways to an income statement, there are many advantages of

BUDGET FORECAST COMPARISON

Company: PTs R US   Income Statement period 1 January 2013 to 31 December 2013

Category	Actual	Budget	Varience	Direction
Gross Sales	36,400	28,400	6,000	F
Less Returns	1,000	400	600	U ✓
Net Sales	35,400	28,000	7,400	F
Purchases	4,000	2,000	2000	U ✓
Cost of Goods Sold	4,000	2,000	2000	U ✓
Gross Profit	31,400	26,000	5,400	F
Interest Income	500	200	300	F
Total Income	31,900	26,200	5,700	F
Salaries	6,500	6,500	0	
Rent	2,300	2,300	0	
Office Supplies	200	300	100	F
Insurance	100	100	0	
Advertising	650	800	150	F
Telephone	300	250	50	U
Travel	500	400	100	U ✓
Total Expenses	10,550	10,650	100	F
Net income	21,350	15,550	+5,800	F

Key: F = favourable U = unfavourable

Figure 19.2 Example budget forecast comparison (for a template visit www.bloomsbury.com/9781408187234)

	Pre-estimate	Jan-07	Feb-07	Mar-07	Apr-07	May-07	Jun-07	Jul-07	Aug-07	Sep-07	Oct-07	Nov-07	Dec-07	Total estimate
Cash on Hand (beginning of month)	5,000	1,570	3,086	4,260	5,705	7,279	9,753	11,128	13,582	16,056	18,631	21,305	23,959	27,584
CASH RECEIPTS														
Cash Sales		1,900	2,000	2,400	2,400	3,300	3,300	3,300	3,300	3,500	3,500	3,500	4,000	
Interest from bank													500	
Loan/ other cash injection														
TOTAL CASH RECEIPTS	0	1,900	2,000	2,400	2,400	3,300	3,300	3,300	3,300	3,500	3,500	3,500	4,500	
Total Cash Available	5,000	3,470	5,086	6,660	8,105	10,579	13,053	14,428	16,882	19,556	22,131	24,805	28,459	27,584
CASH PAID OUT														
Purchases (specify) *1							1,000							1,000
Wages and Taxes			542	542	542	542	542	542	542	542	542	542	542	
Outside services	130			30				20				20		
Rent		192	192	192	192	192	192	192	192	192	192	192	192	
Repairs & maintenance														
Advertising	300			100			100			100			50	
Car, delivery & travel		42	42	42	42	42	42	42	42	42	42	42	42	
Telephone		25	25	25	25	25	25	25	25	25	25	25	25	
Utilities		25	25	25	25	25	25	25	25	25	25	25	25	
Insurance		100												
Interest/bank charges														
Other expenses *2														
Miscellaneous				150										
Accounting & legal														
SUBTOTAL	430	384	826	956	826	826	1,926	846	826	926	826	846	876	1,000
Loan principal payment														
Capital purchase *3	3,000													
Other start-up costs														
Owners' Withdrawal														
TOTAL CASH PAID OUT	3,430	384	826	956	826	826	1,926	846	826	926	826	846	876	1,000
Cash Position (cfwd)	1,570	3,086	4,260	5,705	7,279	9,753	11,128	13,582	16,056	18,631	21,305	23,959	27,584	26,584

*1 items purchased to top up current equipment – also available to sell to clients

*2 any other items purchased to assist in running of business

*3 Initial purchase costs involved in setting up business ie. equipment

Figure 19.5 Example of 12-month cash-flow statement

preparing a cash flow statement (CFS) including the following:

- Indicates areas that use the most cash.
- Which activities generate cash.
- How much is used for investment.
- Comparison to previous years expenditure (same period).
- Indication of debt/credit.

CFSs are often prepared for a year in advance and broken down into monthly periods and identify the sources and amounts of cash coming into a business and the destinations and amounts of cash going out. There are normally two columns, listing forecast and actual amounts respectively. There are many variations of cash flow statements with figure 19.5 showing an example of an annual forecast broken down into monthly periods. It can be seen in the example that in the pre-estimate column that there is a starting (cash on hand) figure of £5,000 which represents an initial start-up cash injection to help the business in the early stages. The CFS then requires a projection of all potential sales income to be entered (see cash receipts), which is difficult for new businesses but can be based on similar periods in previous years for established businesses. Cash receipts cover events such as transfers of cash from other sources or accounts, interest on accounts or borrowing in the form of loans. Once this information is recorded, the total cash available can be calculated by subtracting all the cash receipts from the initial cash on hand figure at the start of each month.

Projections then need to be entered in relation to expenditure (see cash paid out) which when added together give a total cash paid out figure (£3,430 as in the example). Subtracting the total cash paid out from the total cash available then gives the final 'cash position' which is then carried forward to the 'cash on hand' for the following month (£1,570 as in the example). This process is then repeated for each month until a forecast for the whole year has been completed which would result in an annual cash position forecast (£26,584 as in the example). Those new to business may find the amount of financially related information overwhelming; however, there are several principles, known as the 4Ss, which will help the trainer to avoid potential pit-falls.

- **Separate account** – It is important to keep business accounts separate from personal accounts as these will need to be submitted to various agencies and should contain only information that is related to the business.
- **Systems** – No matter how small the transaction it is important to keep records of everything. The success of a business can often depend on the quality and accuracy of its systems, which are also important in the case of audit requirements.
- **Storage** – This refers to the storage of all system information that is generated. If done by computer, make sure back-ups are done regularly and, regardless of the method, make sure everything is stored in accordance with Data Protection guidance. It also refers to getting into the habit of setting up a storage system for receipts even if this just involves categorising and putting them into monthly envelopes.
- **Statement reconciliation** – This is the term used when checking all bank statements to make sure that all recorded transactions can be cross-referenced to appropriate recording sheets and receipts.

APPENDICES

APPENDIX 1: CODE OF ETHICAL PRACTICE

PRINCIPLE 1 – RIGHTS

Fitness Professionals will:

- promote the rights of every individual to participate in exercise, and recognise that people should be treated as individuals
- respect the rights, dignity and worth of every human being and their ultimate right to self-determination. Specifically, exercise professionals must treat everyone equitably and sensitively within the context of their activity and ability – regardless of gender, age, disability, occupation, ethnic origin, colour, cultural background, marital status, sexual orientation, religion or political opinion
- not condone or allow to go unchallenged any form of discrimination, nor to publicly criticise or engage in demeaning descriptions of others
- be discreet in any conversations and refrain from imparting any personal information without consent
- recognise the rights of individuals to confer with other professionals.

PRINCIPLE 2 – RELATIONSHIPS

Fitness Professionals will:

- develop a relationship with their customers based on openness, honesty, mutual trust and respect
- inform participant(s) of their qualifications, experience and registration details and should provide the opportunity for the participant to consent or decline for training/instruction by that person and respect their opinions when making exercise decisions
- not engage in behaviour that constitutes any form of abuse (physical, sexual, motional, neglect, bullying, etc.)
- always promote the welfare and best interests of their participants, and should encourage and guide their customers to accept responsibility for their own behaviour and actions in training and in their relationship with others
- ensure that physical contact is appropriate and necessary and is carried out within recommended guidelines and with the participant's full consent and approval
- avoid sexual intimacy with clients while instructing, or immediately after a training session, and should arrange to transfer the client to another professional if it is clear that an intimate relationship is developing
- take action if they have a concern about the behaviour of an adult towards a child, and must not engage in any form of sexually related contact with minors, including the use of innuendo, flirting or inappropriate gestures and terms
- be aware of the physical needs of people, especially those still growing, and ensure that frequency, intensity, duration and type of training is appropriate

- discuss with parents and other interested parties the potential impact of training programmes offered to minors
- clarify in advance with participants the number of sessions, fees (if any), method of payment, and any other potential costs involved in participation
- if aware of a conflict between their obligation to their customers and their obligation to their trade association, professional institute, the Register or employer must make explicit to all parties concerned the nature of the conflict, and the loyalties and responsibilities involved
- communicate and co-operate with other sports and allied professions in the best interests of their customers. An example of such contact could be the seeking of advice from the British Association of Sport and Exercise Sciences
- communicate and co-operate with registered medical, clinical and ancillary practitioners in the diagnosis, treatment and management of participants' medical, physical and mental problems
- not work with any other professional's customer without first discussing or agreeing both with the professional and customer involved.

PRINCIPLE 3 – PERSONAL RESPONSIBILITIES

Fitness Professionals will:
- demonstrate proper personal behaviour and conduct at all times
- be fair, honest and considerate to all participants and others working in the fitness industry, and will display control, respect, dignity and professionalism
- project an image of health, cleanliness and functional efficiency, and display high stand-ards in use of language, manner, punctuality, preparation and presentation
- not smoke, drink alcohol or use recreational drugs before or while instructing, or to take actions which could compromise the safety of participants
- not adopt practices to accelerate performance or fitness improvements which might jeopardise the safety, total well-being and future participation of their customer(s). Exercise professionals must never advocate or condone the use of prohibited drugs or other banned performance enhancing substances
- ensure that the activities and training programmes they advocate and direct are appropriate for the age, maturity, experience and ability of the participant(s)
- advertise their services with respect to their qualifications, training, knowledge and ability and must be accurate and professionally restrained. They must also be able to present evidence of current qualifications upon request and be able to support any claim associated with the promotion of their services
- have valid public liability insurance cover to adequately and appropriately cover their legal liability in the event of any claim being made
- within the limits of their control, have a responsibility to ensure as far as possible the safety of the participants with whom they work.

PRINCIPLE 4 – PROFESSIONAL STANDARDS

Fitness Professionals will:
- work towards attaining a high level of competence through qualifications and a commitment to ongoing training that ensures safe and

correct practice which will maximise benefits and minimise risks to participants

- promote the execution of safe and effective practice and plan all sessions so that they meet the needs of participants, and are progressive and appropriate
- accept responsibility for their actions, and recognise when it is appropriate to refer to another professional or specialist
- seek to achieve the highest level of qualification available and maintain up-to-date knowledge of technical developments in the fitness industry
- engage in self-analysis and reflection to identify professional needs, and to develop a concept of lifelong learning and personal development
- not assume responsibility for any role for which they are not qualified or prepared
- confine themselves to practise those activities for which their training and competence is recognised by the Register. Training includes the accumulation of knowledge and skills through formal education, independent research and the accumulation of relevant, verifiable experience. The National Occupational Standards for Coaching, Teaching and Instructing (and/or other appropriate fitness awards) provide the framework for assessing competence at the different levels of Register entry. Competence should normally be verified through evidence of qualifications and not inferred solely from evidence of prior experience.
- welcome evaluation of their work by colleagues and be able to account to participants, employers, trade associations, professional bodies and the Register for what they do, and why
- have a responsibility to themselves and their participants to maintain their own effectiveness, resilience and abilities and need to manage their lifestyle to avoid overtraining which might impair performance and cause injury

APPENDIX 2: SUMMARY OF DATA PROTECTION ACT 1998 RELEVANT TO INSTRUCTORS

PART I THE PRINCIPLES

1. Personal data shall be processed fairly and lawfully and, in particular, shall not be processed unless—
   (a) at least one of the conditions in Schedule 2 is met, and
   (b) in the case of sensitive personal data, at least one of the conditions in Schedule 3 is also met.

2. Personal data shall be obtained only for one or more specified and lawful purposes, and shall not be further processed in any manner incompatible with that purpose or those purposes.

3. Personal data shall be adequate, relevant and not excessive in relation to the purpose or purposes for which they are processed.

4. Personal data shall be accurate and, where necessary, kept up to date.

5. Personal data processed for any purpose or purposes shall not be kept for longer than is necessary for that purpose or those purposes.

6. Personal data shall be processed in accordance with the rights of data subjects under this Act.

7. Appropriate technical and organisational measures shall be taken against unauthorised or unlawful processing of personal data and against accidental loss or destruction of, or damage to, personal data.

8. Personal data shall not be transferred to a country or territory outside the European Economic Area unless that country or territory ensures an adequate level of protection for the rights and freedoms of data subjects in relation to the processing of personal data.

APPENDIX 3: GUIDELINES FOR CARDIOVASCULAR MACHINES

Treadmill

Foot action – A heel-toe action should be encouraged at walking and jogging pace as this will help to absorb the shock of impact. At speeds around 8mph, the client should be encouraged to use a mid-foot strike as this will help to eliminate the braking effect.

Arm action – The most efficient way to swing the arms is with a 90 degree angle at the elbows and the arms swinging close the side of the body. Try to keep the shoulders relaxed at all times.

Posture – Encourage the client to maintain a neutral spine with only a slight lean forward, which will increase slightly as the treadmill is inclined.

Cycle
(Upright and recumbent)

Seat height – As the seat height can affect the range of motion and speed of the legs, it is important to make sure that the seat is level with the hip joint of the client when standing next to the cycle (upright only). With the client on the cycle and the feet flat in the pedals, the knee should have a slight bend at the furthest point of the rotation (for both).

Pedal speed (cadence) – Actual pedal speed is dependent on the preference of the client. Most people prefer to pedal between 50 and 80 rpm although this can increase during bouts of high intensity.

Posture – Encourage an upright posture with neutral spine at all times. If using a recumbent cycle, encourage clients not to press the back flat into the seat and to try and maintain a neutral spine.

Stepper

Range of motion – With the whole of the foot placed on the step, encourage a full range of motion that is just before the end range of the machine.

Action – As the leg raises during the stepping, the heel of the same leg should raise slightly of the pedal and return to the pedal as the leg goes down.

Speed – Select a speed that is comfortable for the client. As the level on the step machine is increased, the resistance of the pedals will decrease which means that the client will need to increase the speed.

Posture – Encourage the client to hold the handles just to the side of the body and not out in front. This will enable the client to maintain an upright posture with neutral spine.

Rower

Start position (catch) – With the feet secured in the straps and the knees bent, hold the handle with a pronated grip (overhand) with the arms out straight and a slight bend at the elbows. Keep the wrists straight. The back should be in an upright neutral position.

Drive – Initiate the drive phase with legs pushing out. As the legs are almost at full stretch, pull the handle into the abdomen area.

Recovery – The arms must extend fully before the legs bend to allow the body to come back to the start position. The recovery phase should be twice as long as the drive phase.

Cross trainer

Action – As the leg rises during the stepping action, the heel of the same leg should rise slightly off the pedal and return to the pedal as the leg goes down to mimic actual stepping motion (this helps to promote blood flow round the body as a result of the calf muscle squeezing (venous return).

Range of motion – With the whole of the foot placed on the step, encourage a full range of motion that is just before the end range of the machine.

Posture – Encourage the client to hold the handles to the side of the body and not out in front. This will enable the client to maintain an upright posture with neutral spine.

APPENDIX 4: METHODS OF PREDICTING MAXIMUM HEART RATES

There have been many attempts to find a more accurate calculation for maximum heart rate such as:

- Max heart rate = 206.3 − (0.711 x age); Londeree and Moeschberger
- Max heart rate = 217- (0.85 x age); Miller et al
- Max heart rate (males) = 202 − (0.55 x age); Whyte
- Max heart rate (females) = 216 − (1.09 x age); Whyte

To compound the problems associated with the measurement of maximum heart rate it is generally accepted that it is dependent on exercise type. For instance, studies have shown that maximum heart rate on a treadmill is consistently 5-6 beats higher than on a bicycle ergometer and 2-3 beats higher on a rowing ergometer. It has also been shown that heart rates while swimming are significantly lower, (around 14bpm) than for treadmill running. Research has also shown that elite endurance athletes and moderately trained individuals generally have a maximum heart rate 3 or 4 beats lower than sedentary individuals. For the purpose of designing training programmes at various percentages of heart rate maximum, a combination of the Miller and Londeree and Moeschberger formulas could be used. For example:

Use the Miller formula of MHR = 217 − (0.85 x age) to calculate the MHR of the client, then use the process below to adjust for the specific training method or age of athlete.

Training method or athlete age	Adjustment to maximum heart rate
Treadmill or road running	No adjustment needed.
Rowing	Subtract 3 beats.
Cycling	Subtract 5 beats.
Athletes under 30 years of age	Subtract 3 beats.
50 year old athletes	Add 2 beats.
Athletes over 55 years of age	Add 4 beats.

GLOSSARY

Acetylcholine (Ach) Neurotransmitter substance released from several types of neurones.

Actin Protein structure within a muscle cell.

Active metabolic rate Amount of energy needed over and above a sedentary level.

Adaptation Change due to repeated stimuli such as resistance training.

Adenosine triphosphate (ATP) Main energy currency of the cell.

Adrenalin A neurotransmitter that can stimulate the breakdown of fat and glycogen.

Aerobic In the presence of oxygen.

Aerobic capacity The total amount of energy that can be produced aerobically during a bout of exercise (also known as cardiovascular endurance).

Aerobic fitness The ability to deliver oxygen to the working muscles and use it during exercise.

Amino acid Small molecules that act as the building blocks of any cell needed for growth and repair.

Anaerobic capacity The total amount of energy that can be produced aerobically during a bout of exercise.

Anorexia nervosa An eating disorder characterised by immoderate food restriction and irrational fear of gaining weight.

Agility A rapid whole-body movement with change of velocity or direction in response to a stimulus.

Agonist Refers to a muscle or muscle group responsible for the main action.

Alveoli Air sac in the lungs.

Anaerobic In the absence of oxygen.

Anaerobic fitness The ability to perform maximal intensity exercise.

Anaerobic power The maximal rate at which energy can be produced.

Anaerobic threshold The point at which the energy demand of the exercise being carried out can no longer be met by the aerobic system.

Antagonist Refers to a muscle or muscle group responsible for opposing the main action.

Anthropometry The science relating to the measurement of body mass and proportions of the human body.

Articular cartilage Hard covering on the ends of bones.

Atherosclerosis Narrowing and hardening of the arteries.

Autonomic nervous system Neurons that are not under conscious control.

Axon Branch of a motor neuron.

Basal metabolic rate Rate at which the body uses energy at rest and is measured in Kilocalories.

Blood pressure The force of the blood on the artery walls.

BMI Body mass index (weight/height^2).

Body composition This refers to the ratio of fat to lean tissue in an individual.

Bulimia nervosa Eating disorder characterised by binge eating and purging.

Calorie The amount of energy needed to increase the temperature of 1 gram of water by 1°C.

Cancellous bone A part of a bone that is spongy and contains red marrow.

Capillary The smallest type of blood vessel.

Carbohydrate An organic compound that consists only of carbon, hydrogen, and oxygen.

Cardiac output The amount of blood pumped out of each ventricle per minute.

Cardiovascular disease Disease of the heart (and related vessels).

Cerebral palsy Brain lesions leading to movement and speech problems.

Cholesterol A fat-like steroid used to form cell membranes.

Chondromalacia patellae Injury to the patella due to the femur angle.

Closed Kinetic Chain Exercises in which the body is moving in relation to the load.

Collagen The protein substance of connective tissue.

Compact bone The hard outer layer of a bone.

Concentric contraction A muscular contraction against a resistance in which the muscle length shortens.

Contraction Electrical stimulation of muscle to shorten it.

Contraindications Conditions or circumstances where exercise is contraindicated.

Dehydration Water loss from a state of normal amounts of body water.

Delayed onset muscle soreness Perception of post-exercise soreness.

Developmental stretch A stretch held long enough to induce physical structure development to increase flexibility.

Diaphragm Muscle used to aid breathing.

Diaphysis The shaft of a bone.

Diastasis recti The separation of the linea alba in/following pregnancy.

Diastolic pressure Maximum pressure on the artery walls between contractions of the left ventricle.

Down's syndrome A chromosome disorder which usually causes a delay in physical, intellectual and language development.

Dyslipidemia Abnormal amount of lipids in the blood.

Eccentric contraction A muscular contraction against a resistance in which the muscle lengthens.

EIB: Exercise Induced Bronchoconstriction Difficulty in breathing brought about by exercise.

Emulsification A mixture of two or more liquids that are normally unmixable.

Endocrine system An integrated system of organs, glands and tissues that involve the release of extracellular signalling molecules known as hormones.

Energy The capacity to do work.

Energy system A term used to describe the source or pathway of producing ATP.

Enzymes Proteins that can speed up chemical reactions.

Epicondylitis Inflammation at an epicondyle.

Epimysium Sheath surrounding skeletal muscle.

Epiphysis A region towards the end of a bone known as a 'growth plate'.

Expired air Air that is breathed out.

Extension Movement at a joint in which the joint angle increases.

Extrinsic injury An injury caused as a result of an external force.

Extrinsic motivation The task leads to a reward.

Fascia Type of connective tissue.

Fasciculi Bundle of muscle and nerve fibres bound by connective tissue.

Fast twitch Type of muscle fibre associated with strength and speed.

Flexibility The available range of motion around a specific joint.

Flexion Movement at a joint in which the joint angle decreases.

FEV: Forced expiratory volume in 1 second The volume of air exhaled during the first second of forced expiration.

FVC: Forced vital capacity The volume of air exhaled during a forced maximal exhalation following a forced maximal inhalation.

Gland A group of cells that release hormones.

Glycaemic Index (GI) A ranking of foods from 0–100, based on the rate at which a carbohydrate is broken down

Golgi tendon organs Proprioceptors in tendons sensing force and stretch.

Goniometry Measurement of joint angles.

Haemoglobin Part of a red blood cell that caries oxygen or carbon dioxide.

Heart rate The number of heart beats per minute.

Hemiplegia Full or partial paralysis of one side of the body.

High-density lipoprotein Cholesterol transporters often referred to as the 'good cholesterol' by transporting cholesterol to the liver to be broken down and excreted.

Histamine A chemical in the body that has the effect of widening the airways.

Homeostasis When the systems of the body are working optimally and within normal limits.

Hormone A chemical messenger in the body.

HRmax Maximum heart rate.

Hyperglycaemia High levels of blood glucose.

Hypertension High blood pressure.

Hypertrophy Enlargement of an organ such as muscle.

Hypoglycaemia Low levels of blood glucose.

Hypotension Low blood pressure.

Hypothalamic Relating to the hypothalamus, the part of the brain that regulates the metabolic system.

Hypothermia A body temperature of <34–35°C.

Inspired air Air that is breathed in.

Insulin A hormone secreted by the pancreas, which reduces blood sugar levels.

Intensity A measurement of the difficulty level or 'hardness' of the exercise.

Internal rotation Rotation of a part of the body towards the mid-point.

Intervertebral disc Spongy collagenous disc between vertebrae that acts as a shock absorber.

Intrinsic injury An injury caused as a result of internal forces.

Intrinsic motivation The task itself brings about the reward.

Isokinetic contraction Muscle contraction where the joint angle speed is constant.

Isometric contraction Muscle contraction where there is no change in the muscle length.

Isotonic contraction Muscle contraction against a constant load as in free-weight training.

Ketones Chemicals in the body regarded as toxins.

Ketosis A state where raised levels of ketones are present in the body.

Kyphosis Curvature of the thoracic spine.

Lactic acid A waste product as a result of glycogen breakdown without the presence of oxygen.

Ligament Tissue in the body that connects bone to bone used for support.

Linea alba A band of tendon occurring at the aponeurosis of the abdominal muscles.

Lipid A broad term used for naturally occurring molecules such as fats, waxes and sterols.

Lordosis Excessive primary curve of the lumbar spine.

Low-density lipoprotein Known as the 'bad cholesterol'. Tends to deposit cholesterol on blood vessel walls.

Lumen The channel within a vessel or tube.

Lymphatic system Part of the circulatory system comprising a network of lymphatic vessels that carry lymph (recycled blood plasma).

Metabolic equivalent A method of expressing energy expenditure.

Metabolic rate The amount of energy expended at a given time.

Metabolic syndrome A combination of abdominal obesity, hypertension, dyslipidaemia and impaired fasting glucose.

Mineral A naturally occurring substance that is solid at room temperature.

Mitochondria The 'power cell' or site of aerobic energy production.

Molecule Two or more atoms joined together.

Muscle spindle Structures within muscle that detect changes in length.

Muscular dystrophy A condition that affects muscle fibres and causes weakness. Often results in the use of a powered wheelchair.

Muscular endurance The ability of a muscle or muscle group to perform repeated contractions against a resistance over a period of time.

Muscular strength The maximum amount of force a muscle or muscle group can generate.

Myocardial infarction Irreversible injury to the heart muscle.

Myocardium Essentially the heart muscle.

Myofibril The smallest muscle fibre.

Myosin Protein structure within a muscle cell.

Neural Relating to the nervous system.

Neuromuscular Relating to the muscular and associated nervous system.

Obesity The percentage body fat at which the risk of disease to the individual is increased.

Open kinetic chain Exercises in which the load or resistance is moving in relation to the body.

Origin The attachment point of a muscle to a bone nearest to the midline of the body.

Ossification The process of bone growth.

Osteoblast A bone-building cell.

Osteoclast A bone-modelling cell.

Osteoporosis A condition of reduced bone density.

Outcome goals Goals concerned only with the ultimate outcome.

PAR-Q Physical activity readiness questionnaire.

Pancreas Organ in the body that secretes insulin.

Paraplegia Paralysis of the lower half of the body including the partial or total loss of function of both legs.

Parasympathetic nervous system Division of the autonomic nervous system that can slow the heart rate.

Perceived exertion A subjective measurement of exercise intensity.

Periosteum The tough outer layer of a long bone.

Plyometric Rapid eccentric loading followed by a brief isometric phase and explosive rebound using stored elastic energy and powerful concentric contractions.

POMS/Profile of Mood States Psychological questionnaire used to determine mood states.

Power The product of force and velocity.

Process goals Goals where skills are broken down into manageable units.

Prone Lying on the front.

Proprioception Sense of position in space.

Proprioceptive neuromuscular facilitation A type of stretching.

Protein Chains of individual amino acids

Proximal The segment of the body closest to the centre of the body.

Residual volume The volume of gas remaining in the lungs at the end of a maximal expiration.

Resting heart rate (RHR) The heart rate at resting levels measured in beats per minute (bpm).

RM Repetition maximum

Saccharide Simplest form of carbohydrate.

Sarcomere Unit of contraction in skeletal muscle.

Scoliosis Twisting of the spine.

Self-efficacy Self-confidence in one's ability to succeed.

Skin folds Indirect method of assessing body composition.

Slow twitch Type of muscle fibre associated with endurance.

Smooth muscle Muscle found in the walls of hollow organs that is not under voluntary control.

Stability A body's resistance to the disturbance of equilibrium.

Stretch reflex Reflex action causing contraction within a muscle.

Stroke volume The amount of blood ejected from one ventricle per heartbeat.

Supine Lying on the back.

Sympathetic nervous system Division of the autonomic nervous system, which can speed up the heart rate.

Synergist A muscle or muscle group responsible for assisting the action.

Systolic pressure Maximum pressure on the artery walls during contraction of the left ventricle.

Tendon Connective tissue that surrounds muscle fibres.

Testosterone A hormone that is responsible for muscle growth.

Tidal volume The volume of air that is inhaled or exhaled with each breath.

Tissue A collection of cells with a physiological function.

TLC Total lung capacity.

Transversus abdominis Muscle of the core, involved in forced expiration.

Triglyceride Type of fat used for fuel in the body (glycerol backbone with three fatty acid chains attached).

Validity (test) Purported to specifically measure what the tester or testing team is investigating.

Vasoconstriction Narrowing of the lumen of blood vessels.

Vasodilation Increase in size of lumen of blood vessels.

Vein A vessel that caries blood back to the heart.

Velocity Movement per unit time with direction.

Venous return The amount of blood that enters the heart from the venous circulation.

Vitamin An organic compound required by an organism as a vital nutrient in limited amounts.

Voluntary As a result of conscious thought.

VO_2 The amount of oxygen that is delivered and used by the working muscles ($mlO_2/kg/min$).

VO_2max The maximum amount of oxygen that is delivered and used by the working muscles.

WHR Waist-to-hip ratio.

REFERENCES

American College of Sports Medicine (2009) *ACSM's Exercise management for persons with chronic diseases and disabilities* (3rd ed). Human Kinetics

American College of Sports Medicine (2009) ACSM Guidelines to Exercise Testing and Prescription (8th ed). Lippincott, Williams & Wilkins

Aronson, E., Wilson, T.D. & Akert, R.M. (2003) *Social Psychology*. Prentice Hall

Badland, H. & Schofield, G. (2005) 'Transport, urban design and physical activity: An evidence based update'. *Transport Research* Part D, 10: 177-196

Barasi, M.E. (2003) *Human Nutrition a Health Perspective* (2nd ed). Hodder Arnold

Bean, A. (2006) *The Complete Guide to Sports Nutrition*. A & C Black

Benvenuti, E., Bandinelli, S., Di Iorio, A., Gangemi, S., Camici, S. & Lauretani, F. 'Relationship between motor behaviour in young/middle age and level of physical activity in late life. Is muscle strength the causal pathway?' In Capodaglio, P., & Narici, M.V. (2000) *Advances in Rehabilitation*. PI-ME Press: 17-27

Bettger, F. (1949) How I Raised Myself From Failure To Success In Selling. Prentice-Hall

Blakey, P (2011) *Sport Marketing*. Learning Matters Ltd

Bolton, G (2010) *Reflective Practice: Writing and Professional Development*. Sage

Boreham, C. &, Riddoch, C.J. (2001) 'The physical activity, fitness and health of children'. *Journal of Sports Sciences*, 19: 915–929

British Heart Foundation Health Promotion Research Group (2005) Coronary Heart Disease Statistics. University of Oxford: Department of Public Health

British Heart Foundation National Centre (BHFNC) for Physical Activity and Health. (2012) 'What is sedentary behaviour' Fact sheet, Loughborough University

Brownell, K.D., Stunkard, A.J. & Albaum, J.M. (1980) 'Evaluation and modification of exercise patterns in the natural environment'. *American Journal of Psychiatry*, 137: 1540–1545

Bruce-Low, S. & Smith, D. (2006) 'Explosive exercises in sports training: a critical review. *Journal of Exercise Physiology* online, 9(1):1–10

Chu, L.W., Pei, C.K., Chiu, A., Liu, K., Chu, M.M., Wong, S. & Wong. A. (1999) 'Risk factors for falls in hospitalized older medical patients'. *Journals of Gerontology Series A*, Biological Sciences and Medical Sciences, 54: M38–M43

Curran, S.L., Andrykowski, M.A. & Studts, J.L. (1995) 'Short form of the Profile of Mood States (POMS-SF): Psychometric information'. *Psychological Assessment*, 7(1): 80–83

DEFRA (2001) National Food Survey 2000 Annual report on food expenditure, consumption and nutrient intakes. The Stationery Office

DEFRA (2007) Expenditure and Food Survey 2005-06 Report http://statistics.defra.gov.uk/efs/publications/2006/default.asp

Delozier, M.W. (1978) Marketing communications process. McGraw-Hill

Department of Health (2004) *Choosing Health: Making Healthy Choices Easier*. HMSO

Department of Health (2006) *Health Challenge England: Next Steps for Choosing Health*. HMSO

Department of Health (2006) *Health Survey for England 2006: CVD and Risk Factors Adults, Obesity and Risk Factors Children*. HMSO

Department of Health (1991a) *Dietary Reference Values: A Guide*. The Stationery Office

Department of Health (1991b) 'Dietary Reference Values for food energy and nutrients in the United Kingdom. Report on health and social subjects No.41'. *Report of the Panel of Dietary reference Values of the Committee on Medical Aspects of Food Policy.* The Stationery Office

Department of Health (2011) *Start Active, Stay Active. A Report On Physical Activity For Health From The Four Home Countries' Chief Medical Officers.* The Department of Health

Donaldson, B. (1993) *Sales Management: Theory And Practice.* The Macmillan Press Ltd

Dunnell, K. (2008) *Ageing and mortality in the UK: Population trends 134.* ONS

Egan, G. (1990) *The Skilled Helper.* Brooks-Cole

Epstein, L.H. (1998) 'Integrating theoretical approaches to promote physical activity'. *American Journal of Preventative Medicine,* 15: 257–265

Food Standards Agency (2002) *McCance and Widdowson's The Composition of Foods. Sixth Summary Edition.* Royal Society of Chemistry.

Food Standards Agency (2007) 'Traffic light labelling'. Food Standards Agency Online. http://www.eatwell.gov.uk/foodlabels/trafficlights/

Food Standards Agency (2007) 'The Eatwell Plate'. Food Standards Agency Online. http://www.eatwell.gov.uk/healthydiet/eatwellplate/

Franklin, B.A., Swantek, K.I., Grais, S.L., Johnstone, K.S., Gordon, S. & Timmis, G.C. (1990) 'Field test estimation of maximal oxygen consumption in wheelchair users'. *Archives of Physical Medical Rehabilitation,* 71: 574-578

Gami, A. (2006) 'Secondary prevention of ischaemic cardiac events'. *Clinical Evidence,* (15): 195–228

Glanz, K. & Rimmer, B.K. (1995) *Theory At A Glance: A Guide For Health Promotion Practice.* US Department of Health and Human Services, Public Health Service, National Institutes of Health, and National Cancer Institute

Goulding A. 'Major minerals: calcium and magnesium' in Mann, J. and Truswell, A. S. (eds) (2007) *Essentials of Human Nutrition* (3rd ed). Oxford University Press

Griffin, J.C. (2006) *Client Centered Exercise Prescription* (2nd edition). Champaign: Human Kinetics

Halson, S.L. & Jeukendrup, A.E. (2004) 'Does overtraining exist?: An analysis of overreaching and overtraining research'. *Sports Medicine,* 34: 967–981

Harnirattisai, T. & Johnson, R.A (2005) 'Effectiveness of a behavioural change intervention in Thai elders after knee replacement'. *Nursing Research,* 54(2):97–107

Health Survey for England. (2007) *Healthy Lifestyles: Knowledge, Attitudes and Behaviour.* The NHS Information Centre for Health and Social Care

Health Survey for England 2008. (2009) *Volume 1: Physical activity and Fitness.* The NHS Information Centre for Health and Social Care

Hersey, P. (1988) *Selling a Behavioural Science Approach.* Prentice-Hall

Hoffman, T., Uusitalo-Koskinen, A. & Rusko, H. (1998) 'Variation of athletes' heart rate parameters in the orthostatic test'. *IV Scandinavian Congress on Medicine and Science in Sports,* November 5–8, Lahti: Finland

Hopkins, D. (1993) *A Teacher's Guide to Classroom Research* (2nd ed) The Open University Press

Hynynen, E., Rusko, H., Konttinen, N. & Uusitalo-Koskinen, A. (2003) 'Cardiac autonomic response in overtrained athletes'. *VIIth IOC Olympic World Congress on Sport Sciences,* October 7-11, Athens, Greece: Book of Abstracts, 51B

Janis, I.L. & Mann, L. (1977) *Decision-Making: A Psychological Analysis of Conflict Choice and Commitment.* New York: Collier Macmillan

Joint British Societies (2005) Guidelines on prevention of cardiovascular disease in clinical practice. Heart, 91(V)

Joint Health Surveys Unit (2004) Health Survey for England 2003. Royal Free and University College Medical School: Department of Health

King, A.C., Blair, S.N., Bild, D.E., Dishman, R.K., Dubbert, P.M., Marcus, B.H., Oldridge, N.B., Paffenbarger, R.S. Jr., Powell, K.E. & Yeager, K.K. (1992) 'Determinants of physical activity and interventions in adults'. *Medicine and Science in Sports and Exercise*, 24: S221–S223

Kotler, P. (1997) *Marketing Management: Analysis, Planning, Implementation And Control.* Prentice-Hall

Kotler, P. & Zaltman, G. (1971) 'Social marketing: an approach to planned social change'. *Journal of Marketing*, 35: 3–12

Plisk, S.S. & Stone, M.H. (2003) 'Periodization strategies'. *Strength and Conditioning Journal*, 25: 19–37

Levitt, T. (1967) 'Communications and industrial selling'. *Journal of Marketing*, 31: 15–21

Lockette, K. & Keys, A. (1994) *Conditioning with Physical Disabilities.* Human Kinetics

Londeree, B.R. & Moeschberger, M.L. (1982) 'Effect of age and other factors on HR max'. *Research Quarterly for Exercise and Sport*, 53 (4): 297–304

Marlatt, M.A. & Gordon, J. (1985) *Relapse Prevention.* New York: Guildford Press

McNair, D. M., Lorr, M. & Droppleman, L. F. (1971) *Manual for the Profile of Mood States.* San Diego: Educational and Industrial Testing Services.

Miller, P.D. (1995) *Fitness Programming and Physical Disability.* Champaign: Human Kinetics

Miller, W.C., Wallace, J.P. & Eggert, K.E. (1993) 'Predicting max HR and the HR-VO2 relationship for exercise prescription in obesity'. *Medicine & Science in Sports & Exercise*, 25 (9):1077–1081

Morris, M.H. & Holman, J.L. (1988) 'Source loyalty in organisational markets: a dyactic perspective'. *Journal of Business Research*, 16 (2): 117–131

Narici, M.V. 'Structural and functional adaptations to strength training in the elderly'. In Capodaglio, P. & Narici, M.V. (2000) *Advances in Rehabilitation.* PI-ME Press, 2000: 55-60

National Confidential Enquiry into Patient Outcomes and Death (2009) Caring to the End? A review of the care of patients who died in hospital within four days of admission. NCEPOD

National Institute for Health and Clinical Excellence (2006) 'Obesity: section 2 Identification and classification: evidence statements and reviews'. NICE Clinical Guideline 43. NICE

National Institute for Health and Clinical Excellence (2008) 'Promoting and creating built or natural environments that encourage and support physical activity'. NICE public health guidance 8. NICE

National Institute for Health and Clinical Excellence (2010) 'Lipid Modification: Cardiovascular risk assessment and the modification of blood lipids for the primary and secondary prevention of cardiovascular disease'. NICE Clinical Guideline 67. NICE

NHS Information Centre, Lifestyle Statistics (2009) Statistics on obesity, physical activity and diet: England, February 2009. NHS Information Centre for Health and Social Care

NHS (2006) Statistics on obesity, physical activity and diet: England, 2006. The information Centre, Lifestyle Statistics for Health and Social Care

Office for National Statistics (ONS) (2009a) General household survey 2007: overview, report and data, ONS

Pavlov, I.P. (1927). *Conditioned Reflexes: An Investigation Of The Physiological Activity Of The Cerebral Cortex.* Dover Publications

Peterson, L., Schnor, P. & Sorenson, T.I.A. (2004) 'Longitudinal study of the long-term relationship between physical activity and obesity in adults'. *International Journal of Obesity*, 28: 105–112

Pickton, D. & Broderick, A. (2004) Integrated Marketing Communications (2nd rev ed). Pearson Higher Education

Plisk, J. (2003) 'Principle-based teaching practices'. *National Strength and Conditioning Association Journal*, 25(5): 57–64

Richardson, C., Jull, G., Hodges, P. & Hides, J. (2003) *Therapeutic Exercise for Spinal Segmental Stabilization in Low Back Pain.* Churchill Livingstone

Ross, J.S. & Wilson, J.W. (2006) *Anatomy and Physiology in Health and Illness* (10th ed), Churchill Livingstone

Ross, R., Dagnone, D., Jones, P.J.H., Smith, H., Paddags, A., Hudson, R. & Janssen, I. (2000) 'Reduction in obesity and related comorbid conditions after diet-induced weight loss or exercise-induced weight loss in men'. *Annals of Internal Medicine*, 133(2): 92–103

Ross, R. & Janssen, I. (2001) 'Physical activity, total and regional obesity: dose response considerations'. *Medicine and Science in Sports and Exercise*, 33: S521–S527

Roubenoff, R. & Hughes, V.A. (2000) 'Sarcopenia: current concepts'. *Journals of Gerontology Series A, Biological Sciences and Medical Sciences*, 55: M716–M724

Roy, B.D. (2008) 'Milk: the new sports drink? A review'. *Journal of the International Society of Sports Nutrition*, 5:15

Rusko, H. (2000) 'Overtraining and detection of overtraining by polar heart rate monitors'. 2000 Pre-Olympic Congress, September 7–9, Brisbane: Australia

Schofield, W.N., Schofield, C. & James W.P.T. (1985) 'Basal metabolic rate – review and prediction'. *Human Nutrition: Clinical Nutrition*, 39C(suppl.): 1–96

Sedentary Behaviour Research Network. (2012) 'Standardized use of the terms "sedentary" and "sedentary behaviours"'. *Applied Physiology, Nutrition and Metabolism*. 37: 540–542

Sharkey, B.J. & Gaskill, S.E. (2007) *Fitness and Health*. Human Kinetics

Sheldon, A.F. (1902) The Art of Selling. The Sheldon School

Shirreffs, S.M., Watson, P. & Maughan, R.J. (2007) 'Milk as an effective post-exercise rehydration drink'. *British Journal of Nutrition*, 98: 173–180

Skelton, D.A., Young, A., Greig, C.A. & Malbut, K.E. (1995) 'Effects of resistance training on strength, power, and selected functional abilities of women aged 75 and older'. *Journal of the American Geriatrics Society*, 43: 1081–1087

Stone, W, J. & Klein, D.A. (2004) 'Long-term exercisers: What can we learn from them'. *ACSM'S Health and Fitness Journal*, 8(2): 11-14

Strong, E.K. (1925) *The Psychology of Selling*. McGraw-Hill

Tremblay, A., Almeras, N., Boer, J., Kranenberg, E.K. & Despres, J.P. (1994) 'Diet composition and post-exercise energy balance'. *American Journal of Clinical Nutrition*, 59:975-979

Van Loon, L.J.C., Greenhaff, P.L. & Constantin-Teodosiu, D. (2001) 'The effects of increasing exercise intensity on muscle fuel utilisation in humans'. *Journal of Physiology*, 536: 295–304

Whyte, G.P., George, K., Shave, R., Middleton, N. & Nevill, A.M. (2008) 'Training-induced changes in maximum heart rate'. *International Journal Sports Medicine*, 29(2), p. 129–133

Wilmore, J.H. & Costhill, D.L. (2012) *Physiology of Sport and Exercise* (3rd ed), Human Kinetics

World Health Organization (2002) *The World Health Report 2002. Reducing Risks, Promoting Healthy Life*. WHO Press

World Health Organization. (2005) *The Challenge of Obesity in the WHO European Region and the Strategies for Response*. WHO Press

World Health Organization. (2007) *The World Health Report 2007: A Safer Future: Global Public Health Security in the 21st Century*. WHO Press

World Health Organization. (2000) *ICF: International Classification of Functioning, Disability and Health*. WHO Press

INDEX